PATAÑJALI YŌGA SŪTRA
SAMĀDHI PĀDA

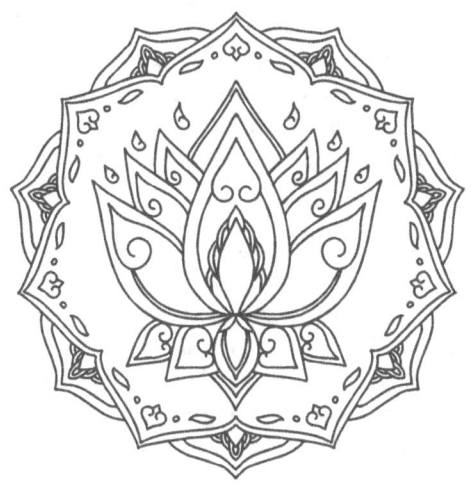

Dr. K.V. Krishnan

Clever Fox®
PUBLISHING
Chennai • Bangalore

CLEVER FOX PUBLISHING
Chennai, India

Published by CLEVER FOX PUBLISHING 2024

ISBN: 978-93-56486-48-5

DEDICATIONS

Ācāryā and lord lakṣmīnrasimhar

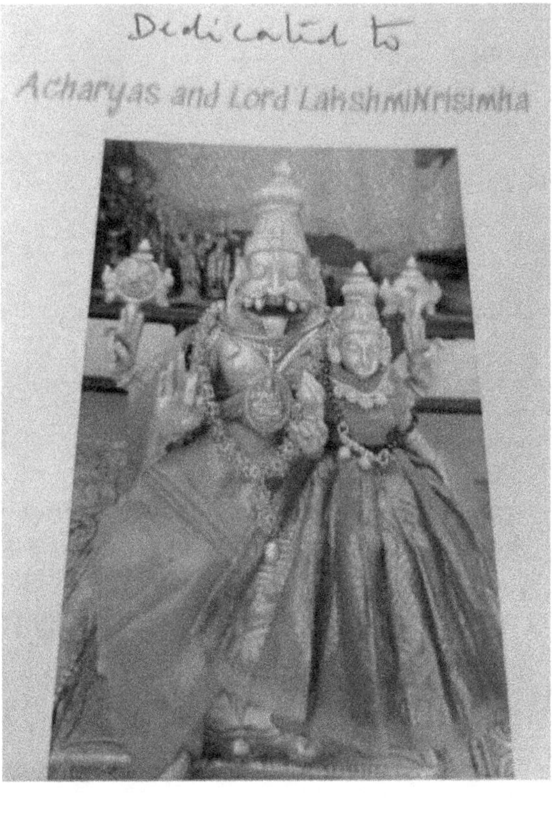

CONTENTS

Foreword v

Acknowledgements vii

Prayer viii

Pride Of Yōgaḥ Sūtrā Granthā x

What is a Sūtra? xv

Introduction 1

Samādhi Pāda 3

Sūtras 4

Bibliography 61

About the Author 62

MAHAJAYAM SPIRITUAL WELFARE TRUST
மகா ஜெயம் ஆன்மீக சமூகசேவை அறக்கட்டளை
Dr.KANDHANADMAI MAHARISHI K R MANDHARACSALAM SWAMIGAL
Palamanallur Road, Bakkothipalayam (Jasmin Kottampatti Village),
Suleeswaranpatti Post, Pollachi, Coimbatore (Dt), Tamilnadu - 642 006.
Phone: 95853 28416, 80720 15790, 98422 56631
Mail id:kandhanadmai@gmail.com Youtube: ASTRO MAHAJAYAM

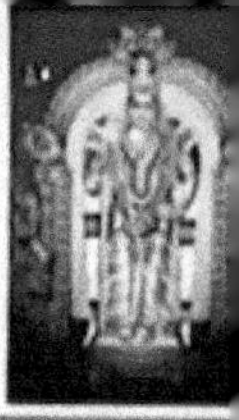

FOREWORD

Date:

15.05.2024

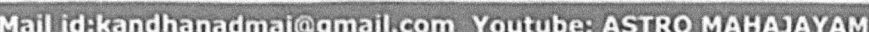

I congratulate Sri. K.V. Krishnan aged 75, on his lucid commentary on the Patañjali Yōga sūtrā

I know him from my Astrology Gurukulam classes. Even at this age, the traditional Yōga he follows during his daily anuṣṭhānā (Rituals) is remarkable. Since I have seen him closely and the way he performs his rituals, makes him a fit candidate to comment about samādhi pāda of Yōga sūtrā by Patañjali Muni. Also due to his knowledge in Sanskrit and Sri Bhāṣyam (the commentary on Brahma sūtrā by Bhagavad Rāmānujā) he is a right candidate for making this commentary on samādhi pāda which is fully about Meditation (dhyāna)

In Hindu philosophy lot of importance is given to meditation and abhyāsa (the practice of Yōga). As far as I know, he follows anuṣṭhānā to the letter and with devotion and so, when he writes a commentary on Yōga sūtrā, it is, referenced from bhāṣyā written by all great Saints and with his own actual experience.

As Hindu tradition says, he has fully followed the sūtrā given by śrī. Patañjali Muni and explanations are made easy and simple for Yōga personnel and youngsters. His commentary is based on Sri Vyāsa bhāṣyam, on Yōga sūtrā and many other scholars such as Vācaspati Miśra, Śaṅkara etc.

He has already written and published two separate books about "Brahma Vidyā"

In that he took the quotes from traditional viśiṣṭādvaitā ācāryā Śrī ālavandār and Sri Bhagavad Rāmānujā. In those volumes he talks about means to attain Liberation through dhyāna and now in this book, he explains (based on Patanjali Muni's Yōga sūtrā), the actual methods for carrying out dhyāna.

I recommend all Yōga personnel and youngsters to read the same and benefit by it.

I wish him all success in his future publications about sanātana dharmā and pray śrī. Lakṣmī nrusimhā to shower His grace on Sri. Krishnan, all the best in his endeavour.

For MAHAJAYAM SPIRITUAL WELFARE TRUST

President

ACKNOWLEDGEMENTS

My sincere Thanks to...

- My Wife Sow Rama

For her moral support and selfless help throughout this effort without which I could not have completed this book

- Mr.S. Sridharan – Advisor, SeniorMentor, and - SeniorYogaTherapist- Kr̥ṣṇamācāri Yōga Manadiram

For his help in proofreading the basic document

- My Long time associate Hemalatha

For her help in formatting the pages

- My daughter Sow. K. Hemamalini

for her ardent help in editing this document and guiding me throughout on book writing

- My Son Chi. K. Madhusudhan

For his encouragement given during preparation of the book

PRAYER

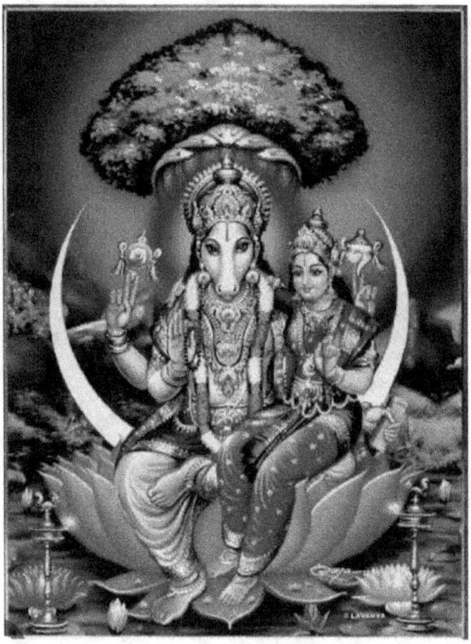

ज्ञानानंदं मयं ददेवं निर्मल स्फटिकाकृतिम्।

आधारं सर्व विद्यानां हयग्रीवं उपास्महे॥

We worship Hayagrīva, whose form embodies pure knowledge and bliss, and who is the foundation of all knowledge, appearing like crystal.

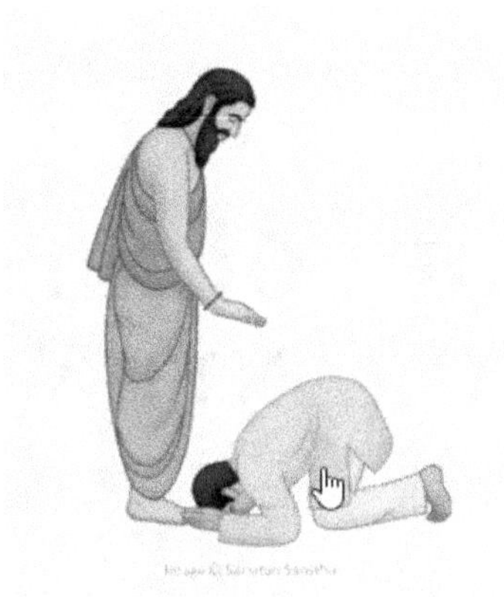

अज्ञान तिमिरान्दस्य ज्ञानाञ्न सलाकया।

चक्षूरुन्मीलितं येन तस्मै श्री गुरुवे नमः।।

Salutations to the revered Guru, by whose grace the darkness of ignorance is dispelled with the torch of knowledge, opening the eyes of wisdom.

गुरुर्ब्रह्मा गुरुर्विष्णुर्
गुरुर्देवो महेश्वरः ।
गुरुस्साक्षात् परं ब्रह्म
तस्मै श्रीगुरवे नमः ॥

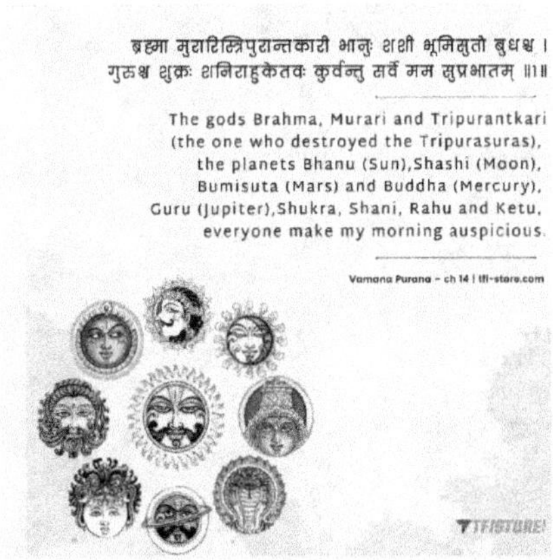

PRIDE OF YŌGAḤ SŪTRĀ GRANTHĀ

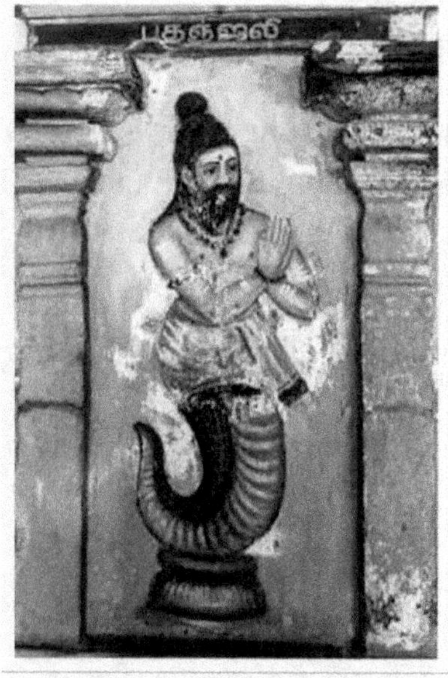

योगेन चित्तस्य पदेन वाचां।

मलं शरीरस्य च वैद्यकेन।

योऽपाकरोत्तं प्रवरं मुनीनां।

पतञ्जलिं प्राञ्जलिरानतोऽस्मि॥

yōgēna cittasya padēna vācām |

malaṁ śarīrasya ca vaidya kēna |

yōpā'karōttaṁ pravaraṁ munīnām |

patañjaliṁ prāñlirānatōsmi ||

yōgēna – through yōgaḥ

chittasya - of the mind

padēna - through speech

vācām - of the words

malaṁ - impurities

śarīrasya - of the body

ca - and

vaidya kēna. - through medicine

yaḥ - who

apā'karōt - removed

taṁ- that

pravaraṁ - excellent

munīnām. - of sages

patañjaliṁ - Patanjali

prāñjalir - with folded hands

anatō- bowed

asmi - I am

I bow with folded hands to patañjali, the best of sages, who removed the impurities of the mind through yōga (**yōga removes impurities of mind**)

Of speech through grammar, and of the body through medicine. These speak volumes of the author who codified the patañjali yōga-sūtrā. we will any way see as we go on. Let us see how he contributed for "speech through grammar"

patañjali means that which fell on an, añjali mudrā in Sanskrit. (pat + añjali) (पत् +अन्जलि) पत् is falling and añjali is a mudrā. So, patañjali as a child, an avatāra of ādhiśēṣa fell in the hands of a lady when she was doing arghya to sun in a river.

Since he was avatāra of ādhiśēṣa, he used to teach sanskrit to his students by taking the form of ādhiśēṣa, with 1000 heads, and used a screen in between him and students. Radiation from ādhiśēṣa would kill them, if the screen is not there.

When he taught the students there was one condition that the screen should never be opened. While, in one session, one boy went out for some reason, others stayed back and out of curiosity they opened the screen. The moment they opened the screen, as was told, they all died. The boy who went out came back to the class later.

patañjali muni was very angry with him and gave śāpa that he would turn into a brahma rākṣas. (**brahma rākṣas are highly intellectual rākṣasā**). The boy pleaded for śāpa vimochana. Out of pity and compassion the muni said. OK, now when you find someone capable to learn Sanskrit grammar, teach that person, at one go entire vyākaraṇa, which I taught in the class (and you have memorised) If you do this successfully, at that time your śāpa will vanish and you will get back your original body.

He asked the student to find such a person. When asked as to how to find such a person, the answer given by Patañjali Muni was as follows.

"Ask the students a question".

Question is "When **tvantam** is added to **pac** the dhātu, how will the word change. Unlike all other words where tvantam is added to the word pac, it turns as पक्व, pac+ tvantam becomes pakva. (पच्+त्वा=पक्व). The śiṣya went on asking the passers-by and at last one boy named vidyādhara answered correctly (out of many who went by) and he was selected and taught the Sanskrit with Grammar by brahma rākṣas for 65 days at a go on top of a pupil tree. This vidyādhara became so tired after 65 days class that he could not even go to the nearest river for a bath. He fell on the way and a lady saved him. This person's son is **vararuci** who later wrote vr̥ttigrantha for pāṇini grammar. vr̥ttigrantha is to edit (add, delete etc) a sūtra text by someone, other than the author but lived in the same time as the sūtra kārar's life. In this incident vararruchi was pāṇini 's classmate and extremely intelligent and so, pāṇini gave him the job of writing vr̥tti over his vyākaraṇa sūtra. **vararuci** learnt Sanskrit grammar through, a śiṣya of Patanjali and so, how he contributed for "speech through grammar" is seen.

None other than vyāsa maharṣi one of the jñāna avatār of lord kr̥ṣṇa Himself wrote bhāṣya for this granthā. In Sanskrit for yōgaḥ, there are many śāstra granthā. In (शतउपनषित्-śata upaniṣat)- one hundred upaniṣad area many are about yōgaḥ. Out of all these the popular one is "patañjali yōga sūtra" śāstra only. There are many vyākaraṇa for the same also.

Some of them are given below:

1. vyāsa bhāṣya by Sri. vyāsa r̥ṣi
   For the above bhāṣya, a vyākaraṇa by vācaspati miśra named tattva vaiśāradhī

2. yoga vārtika by Srivigjanabitchu.
3. rāja mārthānḍam by Sri. Boja raja (a vṛtti grantA)
4. yōga sudhākaram by Sri. sadAsiva brahmendrar-A yōga sūtra vṛtti granthā
5. maṇiprabā by Sri. ramananda yati's vyākaraṇa
6. yōg-siddhānta-candrikā a vyākaraṇa by svāmi nārāyaṇa tīrtar

All these were codified for the welfare of the entire human being. (परोपकारार्थम् इदं शरीरम्)

paropakārārtham idaṁ śarīram, is proved here). Today, this granthā is referred by everyone for any doubt in yōgaḥ

Thus, patañjali yōgaḥ sūtrā passes all requirements of a "pride of a granthā"

WHAT IS A SŪTRA?

अल्पाक्षरं असंदिग्धं सारवत् विश्वतो मुखम् ।

अस्तोभम् अनवद्यं च सूत्रं सूत्रविदो विदुः॥ (वायु पुरान)

alpākṣaram asaṁdigdhaṁ sāravat viśvato mukham.

astobham anavadyaṁ ca sūtraṁ sūtravido viduḥ (vāyu purāna)

अल्पाक्षरं-(alpākṣaraṁ) - few letters

असंदिग्धं-(asaṁdigdhaṁ) - not ambiguous

सारवत्-(sāravat) - essential

विश्वतो-(viśvato) - all sides

मुखम्-(mukham) - mouth

अस्तोभम्-(astobham) - free from defects

अनवद्यं-(anavadyaṁ) - faultless

च-(ca) - and

सूत्रं-(sūtraṁ) - thread

सूत्रविदः-(sūtravidaḥ) - those who know the thread

विदुः-(viduḥ) - know

This verse is from the vāyu purāna. It describes the qualities of a profound truth or principle, Namely, yōgaḥ comparing it to a thread that is simple, clear, pervasive, illumined, and faultless.

A concise, unambiguous knowledge, essential faultless thread, free from defects on all sides, like a moth, and known by those who understand its importance

The essence (sūtraṁ) is few-lettered (simple), not ambiguous, like a thread from all sides (pervading everywhere), with an illumined moth (revealing its meaning), blameless. This sūtra lakṣaṇa was maintained by patañjali muni in yōga sūtra, he wrote.

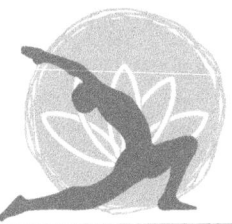

INTRODUCTION

Patañjali muni wrote the following due to great dayā on human beings:

After doing śarīraśuddhi, and obtaining kāya siddhi, and through that, and favourable to this a **vaidya śāstra**, and after doing vāk śuddhi and from that achieve śabda bramha upāsanā to give wellness, and for this **vyākaraṇa of pānini** grammar called mahā bhāṣya, and

To cleanse manas and attain kaivalya, this yōga sūtra

Important attributes are achievements of yōga śāstra are:

1. svarūpa of yōga-sādhana
2. Super natural power one gets as side effects
3. siddhi and kaivalya because of the same (2).

In these matters upaniṣad and yōga śāstra do not have any contradiction. In fact, yogaḥ is a tool to achieve the tatva of upaniṣad and to see them by oneself.

But clashes come because yogaḥ takes sāṅkya śāstra as base. upaniṣad and sāṅkya have many differences, in some important matters and so, yogaḥ and upaniṣad do not agree on certain views.

CHAPTER SUMMARY

sūtra 1,2: Defines yogaḥ

sūtra 3,4: Two possible options for awareness

From sūtra 5 to 11: Description of vṛtti

From sūtra 12 to 16: How to control vṛtti by abhyāsa (practice) and dispassion

sūtra 17,18: Division of samādhi into saṁprajñāta and asaṁprajñāta

sūtra 19: Some discussions on other states that resemble the samādhi

sūtra 20 to 22: How to attain samādhi some pointers

sūtra 23: Introduction of īśvarā and He is the easy method of attaining samādhi

sūtra 24 to 26: īśvarā's nature

sūtra 27 to 29: Chanting īśvarā's name

sūtra 30 and 31: Distractions of manas (Mind) and their accompanying effect.

sūtra 32 to 40: Meditation on any object to combat these distractions

sūtra 41 to 45: Concept of samāpatti and its varities

sūtra 46 to 48: Fruits of samāpatti

sūtra 49: Object of samāpatti, discussion of samāprajñātā - samādhi

sūtra 50, 51: A samāprajñātā samādhi

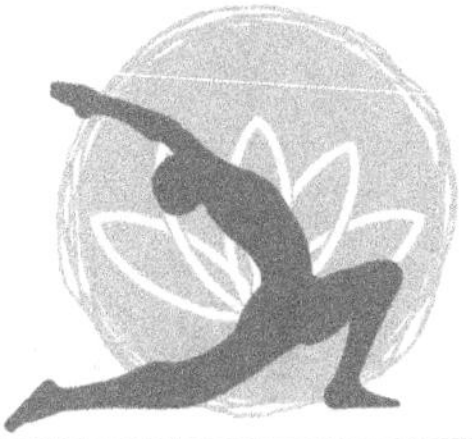

SAMĀDHI PĀDA

समाधिपाद is a term from the ancient Indian philosophical text known as the yoga sūtra, attributed to the sage patañjali

1. समाधि-(samādhi): This word consists of two parts: सम-(sama), meaning "together" or "integrated," and आधि-(ādhi), meaning "mind" or "consciousness." samādhi refers to a state of deep concentration, absorption, or meditative trance, where the mind becomes completely focused and unified.
2. पाद-(pāda): This means "chapter" or "section" in Sanskrit.

   So, समाधि पाद,-translates to chapter on samādhi or section on samādhi and focuses on the state of samādhi, which is considered the goal of **yōga-practice – a state of profound meditative absorption and spiritual realization.**

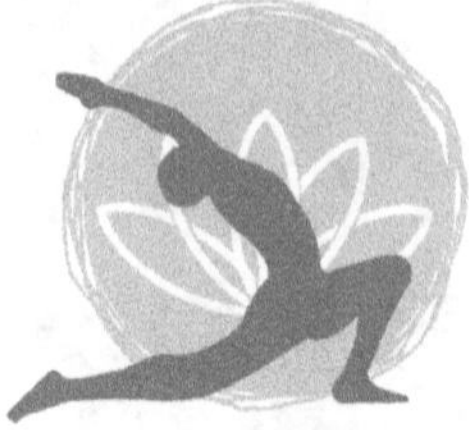

SŪTRAS

अथ योगानुशासनम्।1.1

atha yōgānuśāsanam

योग - yōga

अनुशासनम्-(anuśāsanam) - Instruction or discipline

योगानुशासनम् (yōgānuśāsanam) is a Sanskrit phrase from the yōga-sūtrā of patañjali

This śāstra has been started as told by previous ācāryā.

Now concentration-meditation (the teachings of) is explained.

So, योगानुशासनम् (yōgānuśāsanam) translates to "Instructions on yōga or discipline of yōgaḥ. anuśāsanam in the sūtrā also indicates that patañjali muni has based his yōga-sūtrā on previous śāstrā. He maintained the tradition of old times, kartā for Vedanta was vyāsa and kartā for saṅkhyā was kapila and similarly **kartā for yōgaḥ was hiranya garbar.**

The overall meaning refers to the compilation of teachings and instructions on yōga philosophy and practice, attributed to the sage patañjali. These teachings are foundational in the practice of yōga and provide guidance on various aspects, including ethics, meditation, concentration, and spiritual development

yōgaḥ means samādhi, or to unite. We can also unite jīvā with īśvarā. The author's (patañjali muni's) view is the previous one i.e. samādhi.

patañjali muni has samādhi as the focus point in this granthā. That is to remove jīvā (who has prakr̥ti-saṁbandha) from bandham and make him bandhavimocana (to remove prakr̥ti-saṁbandha). **This is the goal of this granthā.**

citta (Mind-manas) has five stages as given below:

1.	क्षिप्तम्	kṣiptam	oscillations in manas
2.	मूढम्	mūḍham	ignorant state
3.	विक्षिप्तम्	vikṣiptam	for a little time without oscillations in manas, and for long time with oscillations in manas
4.	एकाग्रम्	ēkāgram	focussed on the same vastu
5.	निरुद्धम्	niruddham	This is a state where vr̥tti (Fluctuations, or modifications of the mind-thoughts, emotions, memories, and perceptions in manas) is nil. But only saṁskāra is there.

yogābhyāsa (this is a sanskrit word meaning regular practice of yōga) is not possible in first three states, and in fourth and fifth state it is possible.

योगश्चित्तवृत्तिनिरोधः ।1.2

yōgaścittavr̥ttinirōdhaḥ

yōga is restraining the mind-stuff (citta) from taking various forms (vr̥tti) The mind takes the impression farther in, and presents it to the buddhi – which reacts. The organs (indriyā), together with the mind (manas, buddhi) and egoism (ahamkāra), form the group called the antakaraṇa (the internal instrument). They are various processes in the mind-stuff, called citta. The waves of thought in the citta are called vr̥tti ("the whirlpool" is the literal translation).

What is thought? Thought is a force, as is gravitation or repulsion. It is the mind-stuff, and vr̥ttis are the waves and ripples rising in it when external causes impinge on it. These vr̥ttis are our whole universe.

Further, from this sūtra, it must be noted that nirōdha (the stable asaṁprajñāta- samādhi), alone is yōga is the meaning coming out. "All citta vr̥tti," yogābhyāsa (regular practice of yōga) is not possible, for kṣiptam, mūḍham and vikṣiptam and possible only for other two stated earlier namely ēkāgram, niruddham. Citta is united with sattva, rajas and tamas guṇa. sattva is always with citta, but when it gets associated with rajas and tamas, it attracts all worldly viṣayā - kleṣa

When tamas increases mind is afflicted by adharma, (ajñāna, no-vairāgya, and no-aiśvarya)

When rajas increase, one's mind is afflicted by opposite of kleṣa. when rajas completely decay one can recognise one's true- nature, establishment or stability of one's true nature, namely puruṣa svarūpa pratiṣṭhā. When saṁskāra increases and vr̥ttis decay, it is called asaṁprajñāta samādhi. yōga, is of two types saṁprajñāta samādhi and asaṁprajñāta samādhi. These are respectively also called sa-bījam, nir-bījam.

तथाद्रष्टुः स्वरूपेऽवस्थानम्।1.3

tadā draṣṭuḥ svarūpē'vasthānam

तदा-(tadā): then

द्रष्टु -(draṣṭuḥ): of the seer

स्वरूपे-(svarūpe): in its own form/nature

अवस्थानम्-(avasthānam): state or condition

when this is accomplished (vr̥ttis collapse)- then the seer abides in its own true nature.

When vr̥ttis collapse, there is no viṣayā and that time, puruṣa is in his natural state which is like kaivalya siddhi.

This sūtrā suggests that, through the practice of yōga, one attains a state where the observer or seer realizes its true essence and resides in that state. It reflects the concept of self-realization and understanding one's fundamental nature through the path of yōga

वृत्तिसारूप्यम् इतरत्र।1.4

vr̥ttisārūpyam itaratra.

वृत्ति-(vr̥tti) - fluctuations

सारूप्य-(sārūpya) - identification

इतरत्र-(itaratra) - in other situations (when the mind is not in a state of)

At other times (when one is not in a state of yōga) the seer is absorbed in changing states of the mind. At times other than that of concentration, the yōgi is identified with the modifications. Example, if I am in a state of sorrow, and someone blames me. This is a (vr̥tti or modification) and I identify myself with it and the result is misery.

The overall meaning of this sūtrā is that the yōgi's true nature (sārūpya) is obscured by the modifications of the mind (vṛtti) except in certain states or situations (itaratra). In other words, one's true self is often clouded by the fluctuations of the mind, but in specific circumstances, the true nature can be realized. (True nature is known, when mind is calm without oscillations)

वृत्तयः पञ्चतय्यः क्लिष्टाक्लिष्टाः॥1.5

vṛttayaḥ pañcatayyaḥ kliṣṭākliṣṭāḥ

वृत्तय-(vṛttayaḥ): States, modifications, fluctuation

पञ्चतय्यः-(pañcatayyaḥ): Fivefold

क्लिष्टाः-(kliṣṭā): Painful, afflicted

अक्लिष्टाः-(akliṣṭāḥ): Non-painful, unafflicted

The fluctuations of the mind (changing states of mind) are of five kinds: painful and non-painful. They are either detrimental or non- detrimental to the practice of yōga

This sūtrā describes the various states or modifications of the mind, categorizing them into five types some causing distress or pain (kliṣṭā) and others not causing distress (akliṣṭā). It is a concept of patañjali yōga-sūtrā highlighting the nature of mental fluctuations and their impact on human experience.

प्रमाणविपर्ययविकल्पनिद्रास्मृतयः।1.6

pramāṇa-viparyaya-vikalpa-nidrā-smṛtayaḥ

प्रमाण-(pramāṇa): means of knowledge, proof or source of right knowledge

विपर्यय-(viparyaya) misconception, false
understanding- indiscrimination

विकल्प-(vikalpa) imagination, conceptualization-verbal delusion

निद्रा-(nidrā): sleep

स्मृतयः-(smṛtayaḥ): memories

The sūtrā suggests that our vṛtti (mental activities) can be categorized into five types -

pramāṇa (correct knowledge), viparyaya (misconception, error), vikalpa (imagination), nidrā (sleep), and smṛti (memory)

प्रत्यक्षानुमानागमाः प्रमाणानि।1.7

pratyakṣānumānāgamāḥ pramāṇāni

प्रत्यक्ष-(pratyakṣa): Perception, direct observation

अनुमान-(anumānā): Inference

आगमाः-(āgamāḥ): Testimony, authoritative statement

प्रमाणानि-(pramāṇāni): Means of valid knowledge or sources of knowledge

Right knowledge consists of sense perception, (inference)-logic, and authoritative or competent verbal testimony

This sūtrā, conveys the same idea as the previous one, highlighting the three traditional sources of valid knowledge in Sanatana-philosophy: direct-sense perception, inference, and testimony.

आगमाः (Testimony) is, testimony from reliable sources, (given by jñānis, munis etc,.) śabda, and īśvara's vācakam. There are differences in these three pramāṇā.

Ordinary persons take pratyakṣa as pramāṇā. A person with little more intellect and jñāna takes pratyakṣa and anumānā as pramāṇā. A person with much more jñāna takes śabda also as pramāṇā. All these pramāṇā are only till one attains ātmasātkṣātkāra. Post this ātmasātkṣātkāra, that itself (only) is the pramāṇā. To attain that highest state only these pramāṇā are required (they act as ladder) and are sādhanā

विपर्ययो मिथ्याज्ञानम् अतद्रूपप्रतिष्टम्।1.8

viparyayō mithyājñānam atadrūpapratiṣṭham

विपर्यय: -(viparyayaḥ) - misconception or misunderstanding

मिथ्या-(mithyā) - false or incorrect

ज्ञानम्-(jñānam) - knowledge

अतत्-(atat) - not of that form

रूप-(rūpa)-form

प्रतिष्टम्-(pratiṣṭham) – established in

Error, false knowledge which stems from incorrect apprehension. Indiscrimination is false knowledge, not established in real nature, mistaking one thing for another.

viparyaya is a matter appearing in a false and different svarūpa instead of actual one of the matters.

Doubt is a part of viparyaya is the thinking of the sage patañjali

शब्दज्ञानानुपाती वस्तुशून्यो विकल्पः।1.9

Śabda jñānanupātī vastu śūnyō vikalpaḥ

शब्द-(śabda)-words, sound

ज्ञानान-(jñāna)-knowledge

अनुपाती –(anupātī)-resulting from,

वस्तु- (vastu)-actual object

शून्य: -(śūnyaḥ)-devoid of

विकल्पः-(vikalpaḥ)-fancy, imagination or conceptualization.

Imagination consists of the usage of words that are devoid of an actual object

The term suggests that vikalpa (conceptualization or alternative thoughts) arises from the knowledge of words when it is not grounded in real substance or objects. It points towards the idea that mental constructs can be divorced from actual reality, when they are based solely on language or words without a corresponding reality. Therefore, one must learn from a guru and not from books and **"I think I know"**

vikalpaḥ- is matter is not there really but a mind's vr̥tti (mano vr̥tti) based on a word alone.

अभावप्रत्ययालम्बना वृत्तिर्निद्रा।1.10

abhāvapratyayālambanā vr̥ttirnidrā.

अभाव-(abhāva)- absence

प्रत्यय-(pratyaya)-mental modification

आलम्बन-(ālambanā)- supported by

वृत्ति-(vr̥tti)- state of the mind, mental activity or modification

निद्रा-(nidrā)- sleep

Deep sleep (nidrā) is that state of mind which is devoid of any modifications or absence of any content.

The overall meaning of this sūtrā is that sleep (nidrā) is a mental state where the mind is devoid of any modifications or mental activities. It is a state characterized by the absence of mental fluctuations or modifications.

The next class of vr̥tti is called sleep and dream. sleep is a vr̥tti which embraces the feeling of voidness. Sleep is when outside viṣaya prajñā is absent and sattva, rajas guṇa are less and tamas guṇa is of high nature and associated with avidyā. When, we are awake, we know that we have been sleeping; we can only have memory of perception. That which we do not perceive we never can have any memory of. Every reaction is a wave in the lake. Now, if, during sleep, the mind has no waves, it would have no perceptions, positive or negative, and, therefore, we would not remember them. The very reason of our remembering sleep is that during sleep there was a certain class of waves in the mind. Memory is another class of vr̥tti which is called smr̥ti

अनुभूतविषयासंप्रमोषः स्मृतिः ।1.11

anubhūtaviṣayāsaṁpramōṣaḥ smr̥tiḥ

अनुभूत-(anubhūta)-experienced

विषय-(viṣaya)-object

असंप्रमोषः-(asaṃpramoṣaḥ)-losing hold

स्मृतिः-(smr̥tiḥ) memory-recollection

Memory is retention of images of sense objects that have been experienced.

Memory is the recollection of experienced objects when the hold or impression of those objects has faded away. This sūtrā suggests that memory involves recalling past experiences when the vividness or impact of the objects of those experiences has diminished or faded.

smṛti is experienced viṣayā does not leave the manas. One who has experienced the vr̥tti through pramāṇā is because of sukha duḥkha moha. Out of these, pramāṇā, viparyayaḥ, and vikalpaḥ are experienced when one is awake.

Only vāsana is experienced in swapna avasthā. nidrā is in suṣupthi avasthā alone. smṛti is not in nidrā but in other two avasthā

अभ्यासवैराग्याभ्यां तन्निरोधः।1.12

abhyāsavairāgyābhyāṁ tannirōdhaḥ

अभ्यास-(abhyāsa)-Practice

वैराग्याभ्यां-(vairāgyābhyāṁ)- dispassion, renunciation, detachment or non-attachment

तत्-(Tat)-Their, that vṛtti state of mind

नरोिधः(nirōdhaḥ)- Control or Restraint

The vritti state of mind is stilled by practice and dispassion.

The overall meaning of this sūtrā is that control of the mind can be achieved through the consistent practice (abhyāsa) and detachment (vairāgya). It suggests that cultivating a balance between disciplined practice and non-attachment can lead to mental control and stillness. The vṛttis seen above can be controlled (nirōdhaḥ) by means of abhyāsa and vairāgya.

तत्र स्तितौ यत्नोऽभ्यासः।1.13

tatra stitau yatnō'bhyāsaḥ

तत्र-(tatra)-of these

स्थितौ-(sthitau)- in the matter of steadfastness

यत्नः-(yatnaḥ)- effort

अभ्यासः-(abhyāsaḥ)- practice

अभ्यासः– (abhyāsaḥ) **-Practice is the effort fixed in concentrating the mind**

Effort is there in being situated there (as potential). This could imply the importance of consistent practice or effort (we must manifest the same) in a particular place or situation.

Abhyāsa is to keep the manas stable and steady in puruṣa

स तु धीर्गकाल नैरन्तर्यसत्कारासेवितो दृढभूमिः।1.14

sa tu dhīrgakāla nairantaryasatkārāsēvitō dṛḍhabhūmiḥ

सः–(saḥ)- it, practice

तु –(tu)- but

धीर्गकाल –(dhīrgakāla)- prolonged period of time

नैरन्तर्य-(nairantarya)- uninterruptedly

सत्कार-(satkāra)- with reverence

असेवितः-(asevitaḥ)- attended or served, practiced

दृढ-(dṛḍha)-firm

भूमिः–(bhūmiḥ)-ground, with firm determination or unwavering mind

Abhyāsa (practice) becomes firmly established when it has been cultivated uninterruptedly with devotion and great effort for a prolonged period on a specific lakṣya

दृष्टानुश्रविकविषयवितृष्णस्य वशीकारसंज्ञा वैराग्यम्।1.15

dṛṣṭānuśravikaviṣayavitṛṣṇasya vaśīkārasaṁjñā vairāgyam.

दृष्टा-(dṛṣṭā)-visible, perceptible

अनुश्रविक-(anuśravika)- heard about from scripture

विषय-(viṣaya)-sensual objects

वितृष्णस्य-(vitṛṣṇasya) – from one who is free from craving

वशीकार-(vaśīkāra)-subdue, exert control

संज्ञा-(saṁjñā) – consciousness,

वैराग्यम्-(vairāgyam) – renunciation, dispassion

Dispassion(vairāgya) is the controlled conscious state of one who is without craving for sense objects whether perceived or described in scriptures.

Vairāgya is- leaving to itself pratyakṣā, and apratyakṣā viṣaya without desire or interest in the same

Desire to leave or non-desire in viṣaya is Vairāgya. This has four steps.

1. **yatamānam** - effort to prevent manas from going to senses.
2. **vyatirekam** - this is, to know the differences in viṣaya, i.e. Some of them though left by us will still try to attract us towards them. We have not started any preventing action for the same. On these we must develop Vairāgya and leave them.
3. **ekendriyam**-Third step is, to avoid senses becoming averse to this Vairāgya on viṣaya already left by us, practice manas alone to like or dislike them. Since manas indriya still involved it is called ekendriya.
4. **vaśīkarā** -All viṣaya vanishes by these efforts. Senses are not averse. Likes, dislikes also get out of manas. Hence now instead of Indriya under control of viṣaya, viṣaya is controlled by indriya. This happens by puruṣa darśana. See BG sloka below:

विषया विनिवर्तन्ते निराहारस्य देहिनः।

रसवर्जं रसोऽप्यस्य परं दृष्ट्वा निवर्तते।।(BG 2.59)

One may restrain the senses from their objects of enjoyment, but the taste for the sense objects remains. However, even this taste ceases for those (a yōgi) who realizes the Supreme.

तत्परं पुरुषख्यातेर्गुणवैतृष्ण्यम्।1.16

tatparaṁ puruṣakhyātērguṇavaitṛṣyam

तत्परं- (Tat-param) – That-higher

पुरुष-(puruṣa)-soul, self

ख्याते:(khyāteḥ) - of the knowledge or perception of the person

गुण-(guṇa)-qualities of sattva, rajas and tamas

वैतृष्ण्यम्-(vaitṛṣṇyam) – indifference, freedom from craving for qualities

Higher than renunciation is indifference to guṇa which comes from perception of the puruṣa (soul)

The overall meaning of this sūtrā can be interpreted as the state of liberation or enlightenment where an individual is no longer attached or craving for the qualities or attributes of the external world, having attained supreme knowledge or realization of the self.

That extreme non-attachment, giving up even the qualities, shows (the real nature of the puruṣa).

It is the highest manifestation of power when it takes away even our attraction towards the qualities. We have first to understand what the puruṣa, the self, is, and what are its dormant qualities which can manifest if we realise.

According to yōga-philosophy, the whole of nature consists of three qualities – one is called tamas, other rajas and the third sattva. These three qualities manifest themselves in the physical world as attraction, repulsion, and control.

Everything that is in nature, (all these manifestations) are combinations and recombinations of these three forces. The self of man is beyond all these, beyond nature, and is effulgent by its very nature. It is pure and perfect.

The self of man (ātmā) is beyond all these, beyond nature, is effulgent by its very nature. It is pure and perfect. Whatever, of intelligence we see in nature is but the reflection from this self upon nature. Nature itself is insentient. One must remember that the word nature also includes the mind; mind is in nature; thought is in nature; from thought, down to the grossest form the self of man is beyond all these, beyond nature, is effulgent by its very nature. It is pure and perfect. The self of man is beyond all these, beyond nature, is effulgent by its very nature. It is pure and perfect.

sādhāraṇa (ordinary) vairāgya is not having attachment to the cause of which is kārya.

parama vairāgya means and is because of puruṣa darśana and not having attachment to viṣaya, sattva, rajas, and tamas guṇa. sādhāraṇa (ordinary) vairāgya is when sattva guṇa is increased and associated with rajas but having no tamas guṇa. In this one can attain siddhi, one can get svarga, prakṛtilayā, videhi sthiti. But one who has parama vairāgya (a yōgi) even though can experience everything (anubhava), he is indifferent to viṣaya, and having a goal for puruṣa darśana, does ātma sātsākṣkāra

वितर्कविचारानन्दास्मितारूपानुगमात् संप्रज्ञातः ।1.17

vitarkavicārānandāsmitārūpānugamāt saṁprajñātaḥ

वितर्क-(vitarka): absorption with physical awareness

विचार-(vicārā)- absorption with subtle awareness

आनन्द-(ānanda)- absorption with bliss

अस्मिता-(asmita)- absorption with sense of "I" ness

रूप-(rūpa)-form

अनुगमात्-(ānugamāt)- accompanied by

संप्रज्ञातः-(saṁprajñātaḥ)- samādhi state which still uses manas and an object for meditation

saṁprajñāta- samādhi- consists of consecutive mental state of absorption with physical (vitarka) awareness, absorption with subtle awareness (vicārā), absorption with bliss(ānanda), absorption with sense of "I" ness (ānanda)

First sādhana and then sādhya namely samādhi. is spoken by patañjali muni. samādhi. is of two types;

first is saṁprajñāta samādhi and second is asaṁprajñāta samādhi.

saṁprajñāta samādhi has four internal divisions: vitarka, vicārā, ananda, asmitā

A yōgi

first does dhyana on a sthūla vastu- **vitarka**

next he does dhyana on the sūkṣma of the vastu namely tanmātrā - **vicārā**

next preventing indriya from going after sthūla vastu and practices to stay where it is by which one gets an anubhava - **ananda.**

Asmitā- By prayatna block anything else coming into mind and only "I" ness (prajñā) stays in him- Vicārā, ānanda, asmita are in vitarka. Ananda and asmita are in vicārā. asmita alone is in ananda. In this method mind seizes something (anubhava) and that is why it is saṁprajñāta samādhi

विराम प्रत्यय अभ्यासपूर्वः संस्कार शेषः अन्यः।1.18

virāma pratyaya abhyāsapūrvaḥ saṁskāra śēṣaḥ anyaḥ

विराम-(Virāma)-cessation

प्रत्यय-(pratyaya)-mental modifications or thoughts

अभ्यास-(abhyāsa)-practice

पूर्वः-(pūrvaḥ)-previous

संस्कार-(samskāra)-impressions

शेषः-(śēṣaḥ)-residue

अन्यः(anyaḥ)-other

asaṁprajñāta- samādhi- is determination to terminate past impressions- (all thoughts). In this state, only latent impressions remain.

Once abhyāsa of this method become stable (stira), mind stays alone without any ālaṁbana (support). But saṁskāra śeṣam (fulfilment of various rituals or ceremonies such as birth, marriage, death, will be there during this state) This will also vanish when this samādhi is stable. This state is when all vr̥tti have gone. Only prajñā exists. It is like an ocean without waves. rajas and tamas will not be there and it would become sattva-guna svarūpa. parama vairāgya is the means for this higher state. Manas in ēkāgram (undisturbed or concentrated) state is when **saṁprajñāta- samādhi happens.**

भवप्रत्ययो विदेहप्रकृतिलयानाम्।1.19

bhavapratyayō vidēhaprakr̥tilayānām

भव-(bhava)-becoming

प्रत्यय: -(pratyayaḥ)- with material existence, cause, the apprehension of existence, the thought pattern arising from identification

विदेह-(Videha) Devoid of a gross body, unembodied

प्रकृति-लयानाम्-(Prakṛtilayānām) absorption into nature, merging with the material world (matter)

This means only by detachment to worldly pleasures one can overcome cycles of birth

This sūtrā suggests that the thought patterns or mental impressions arising from identification with material existence cease when one becomes disembodied or transcends physicality. It implies that through detachment from the physical body and absorption into nature, one can overcome the cycles of worldly existence and attain higher states of consciousness. The state of saṁprajñāta- samādhi is characterised.

This samādhi when not followed by extreme detachment becomes the cause of remanifestation

of those that merge with nature.

This asaṁprajñāta- samādhi, when vairāgya is not fully attained gives dēva-sthāna and prakr̥ti-laya sthāna

asaṁprajñāta- samādhi has two types.

bhavapratyaya- (a state where impressions or residual tendencies known as saṁskāra - exist and these impressions can potentially influence future thoughts and actions and a yōgi tries to transcend even these subtle impressions to achieve highest state of meditative absorption)

The cause for this is avidyā. yōgi in this state will have desire to have bogam (enjoy) of many bhuvana. This state has time limitations. vāyupurāṇa, describe these time limitations. Those who do upāsana of mahat and avyaktam and do upāsana that self and they are one and the same, gets laya with vastu post death (after śarīra falls)

upāya pratyaya

the use of manas is to get (give) only puruṣa sātkṣātkāra. If manas does not have interest in prakr̥ti laya anubhava stated above, and concentrates and gets puruṣa sātkṣātkāra, that is called kaivalya state. This is what is known as **upāya pratyaya.** Those who do upāsana of mahat (buddhi) as self will continue to live in this bhuvana for 10,000 manvantarā. and those who do upāsana on avyaktam live for 100,000 manvantarā and those who get puruṣa sātkṣātkāra, upāsana that self and they are one and the same, transcends time is stated in vāyupurāṇa

श्रद्धावीर्यस्मृतिसमाधिप्रज्ञापूर्वक इतरेषाम्।1.20

śraddhāvīryasmr̥tisamādhiprajñāpūrvaka itarēṣām

श्रद्धा-(śraddhā)-Faith

वीर्य-(vīrya)-Energy, vigor

स्मृति-(smr̥ti)-Memory

समाधि-(samādhi)-absorption, Contemplation

प्रज्ञा-(prajñā)–discernment, Wisdom

पूर्वक-(pūrvaka)-preceded

इतरेषाम्-(itarēṣām) –for others

For others (for those only sub-conscious impressions remain) this samadhi is preceded by faith, energy, memory, samādhi, and (discernment)-wisdom.

Whatever was stated earlier, is not considered by others (such as stana (stiti) of dēva, prakṛti laya-sthāna), get kaivalya through śraddhā, vīrya, smṛti, prajñā and samādhi.

In these, **śraddhā** is the clarity of manas to attain the higher stiti of kaivalya and because of this special-efforts by manas.

vīrya is to have better clarity of buddhi

smṛti is to keep thinking of above stated efforts to attain kaivalya

prajñā is manas to attain samādhi, and to have real experience

samādhi is to attain niścalam ēkāgriyam of manas

important point is that each step depends on attaining the previous step

तीव्रसंवेगानाम् आसन्नः ।1.21

tīvrasaṁvēgānām āsannaḥ

तीव्र-(tīvra)-intense

संवेगानाम्-(saṁvegānām)-impetus or fervour

आसन्नः-(āsannaḥ)-approaching or close to

This state of saṁprajñāta is near for them who apply themselves intensely. The verdict is saṁprajñāta samādhi's phala is asaṁprajñāta samādhi. asaṁprajñāta samādhi's phala is kaivalya.

For those who have tīvra (intense)-vairāgya (aversion to viṣaya), the samādhi state is very near

yōgis follow nine steps. They vary because of differences in upāya (means) and vairāgya (aversion to viṣaya)

upāya is of three types, mr̥du, madhyama, adhimātra. A yōgi who has adhimātra vairāgya, sees samādhi state very near as stated in this sūtra. They get samādhi lābha samādhi bala

Why everyone even-though they apply śraddhā do not get samādhi easily is due to differences in upāya and vairāgya and this is due to previous birth's samskāra viśēṣa

मृदुमध्याधिमात्रत्वात् ततोऽपि विशेष:।1.22

mr̥dumadhyādhi mātratvāt tatō'pi viśeṣaḥ

मृदु-(mṛdu)-mild

मध्य-(madhya)-moderate

अधिमात्रत्वात्-intense

ततः-(tataḥ)-from this consequently, therefore

अपि-(api) -also

विशेष: -(viśeṣaḥ)-particularly or especially, distinction

Even among these, there is further differentiation of this intensity into mild, mediocre, and extreme. saṁprajñāta-samādhi is a term used in yōga-philosophy to describe a state of meditation characterized by conscious awareness and mental focus. It is often translated as "conscious" or "discriminative" meditation.

In saṁprajñāta-samādhi, the practitioner maintains awareness of the object of meditation along with the process of meditation itself. This state involves a clear and focused mind, where there is still some level of mental activity and awareness of the self

It is contrasted with asaṁprajñāta-samādhi, which is a state of meditation without any mental activity or awareness of objects, often described as "unconscious" or "non-discriminative" meditation. This is the state a yōgi wants to reach.

ईश्वरप्रणिधानाद् वा ।1.23

īśvarapraṇidhānād vā

ईश्वर-(īśvara) means "Lord" or "Supreme Being."

प्रणिधानाद्-(praṇidhānād)-dedication, devotion, or surrender.

वा-(vā)-or

Or, (this previously mentioned state is attainable) from devotion to the īśvara

This phrase suggests the importance of surrendering to or dedicating oneself to īśvara, implying the value of humility, faith, and submission to a higher power in one's spiritual practice or life journey.

Also, this suggests previously mentioned state is attainable through devotion or surrender to īśvara

The discussion here is " is there a way to liberation other than the two mentioned here". abhyāsa or vairāgya?

Yes, may be through devotion or surrender. īśvara alone and nothing else is aimed at in withdrawal from worldly affair and therefore focus on knowledge about bramhan.

This is not tenable. Practice or dispassion cannot be optional. Therefore "va" of the sūtrā must be read as self-reliance to previous sūtrā 1.20 to 1.22. namely apply faith, vigour, memory, samādhi, by self or surrender with devotion to īśvara

Īśvara bakti is special viśēṣa

īśvarapraṇidhānā is one can get samādhi lābha by pure affection to Īśvara

without any other thoughts only by pure affection (devotion) to Īśvara this siddhi of samādhi-lābha

is achieved. bhakti happens through manas, vāk and kāya. See what BG has to say on this.

अनन्याश्चिन्तयन्तो मां ये जनाः पर्युपासते।

तेषां नित्याभियुक्तानां योगक्षेमं वहाम्यहम् ।। BG 9.22

वहामि - I carry

And the overall meaning of this verse is:

"For those who constantly worship Me with exclusive devotion, meditating on My transcendental form, I preserve what they have and carry what they lack.

Īśvara promises to CARRY OUR burden. He does not say I will take care etc., but carry is a very strong word.

क्लेशकर्मविपाकाशयैर्परामृष्टः पुरुषविशेष ईश्वरः।1.24

klēśakarmavipākāśayairparāmṛṣṭaḥ puruṣaviśēṣ īśvaraḥ

क्लेश-(kleśa)-afflictions, pains, obstacles to practice of yoga

कर्म-(karma)-actions, deeds

विपाक-(vipāka)-fruitition, maturing, consequences

आशयैर्-(āśayair)-storehouse, accumulation

अपरामृष्टः-(aparāmṛṣṭaḥ)-untouched

पुरुष-(puruṣa)-individual, person, soul

विशेष-(viśeṣa)-particular, special

ईश्वरः-(īśvaraḥ)-supreme being, Lord

The Bramhan is a special soul. He is untouched by obstacles, to the practice of yōga, karma, and subconscious predispositions. The supreme being (īśvaraḥ) is a special puruṣa,untouched by afflictions (kleśa) to the practice of yōga, actions (karma), fruits of actions (vipāka), and (āśayair- vāsanā)

klēṣa is- rāga, dvēśa, avidyā, and abhinivēśa

karma is the cause of these the pava and punya

phala is that karma's effect (result)

āśaya is pūrva karma vāsanā. These only are reasons for any action(karma) in this birth. This is in **citta** in the form of samskāra. Since a puruṣa enjoys their results, these get into him.

īśvaraḥ is one who does not attract any of these bōga (pleasure or enjoyment)

In buvana, there are **no** two-vastus identical in all aspects. At-lest **by time** they would be different. The difference between mōkṣa by advaita and kaivalya by yōgis is, that in in mōkṣa by-advaita bedam (difference) will not be there between jīva(puruṣa) and **īśvaraḥ,** and attaining akaṇṭaka vṛtti after bedam vanishes is moksha. But, in kaivalya **īśvaraḥ** and Jiva Bedam (separate concept) exists.

īśvaraḥ's citta dissolves in prakṛti during pralaya.

तत्र निरतिशायं सर्वज्ञबीजम्।1.25

tatra niratiśāyāṁ sarvajña bījam

तत्र-(tatra)- in Him, there

निरतिशायं-(niratiśāyāṁ)-unparalleled, unsurpassed

सर्वज्ञ(sarvajña)-omniscience

बीजम्-(bījam)-seed

In him the seed of omniscience is unsurpassed. Pleasure and pain are one's own result of one's own past actions and has nothing to do with īśvaraḥ

īśvaraḥ's sarvajñatvam (omniscience) is unsurpassed

śankarā said" īśvaraḥ is pure sattva and so free of limitations of conventional bodies. Therefore,

īśvaraḥ's awareness can be simultaneously in contact with everything that is omniscient.

īśvaraḥ has a shakti to know everything simultaneously

पूर्वेषाम् अपि गुरुः कालेनानवचछेदात्।1.26

pūrvēśām api guruḥ kālēnānavacchēdāt

पूर्वेषाम्-(pūrveṣām) - of the ancients, of those who have gone before

अपि-(api) - also, even

गुरुः-(guruḥ) - a teacher, a master

कालेन-(kālena) - by time, with time

अनवच्छेदात्-(anavacchedāt) - without limitation, without obstruction

Even the masters of the past were not exempt from the passage of time including īśvaraḥ since He was also the teacher of ancients. Since īśvaraḥ is beyond time, He is the guru of all gurus.

īśvaraḥ has special śakti to know everything simultaneously without interruption.

Many examples could be given from purāṇa to show this point.

Even caturmukha brahmā was taught the entire veda by īśvaraḥ and advised him to make vyaṣṭiśruṣṭi as it was before. (Brahman makes the twenty-four śriṣṭis first and then brahmā takes over again with the help of (bramhan)

Although He has nothing to achieve for Himself, His motivation to benefit the living beings is

His compassion for them: He "instructs the living beings of saṁsāra dharma -knowledge through veda, that is how He delivers them. He is the guru even of the gurus of the

past as He is not limited by time.

Īśvaraḥ is jñāna svarūpi. When jñāna expands and the place where it ends is said to be īśvaraḥ, one can think that īśvaraḥ, exists. The question then is why do we need śabda pramāṇa? Because the knowledge comes that īśvaraḥ, exists by this method, only sāmānya jñāna only without His guṇa viśēṣa will be activated. But śabda pramāṇa gives full knowledge including guṇa viśēṣa

तस्य वाचक: प्रणवः I1.27

tasya vācaka: praṇavaḥ

This "om " is a mystical syllable and designates the bramhan.

तस्य- (tasya) - his/its

वाचकः-(vācakaḥ) - indicating, denoting, representing

प्रणवः-(praṇavaḥ) - the sacred syllable oṁ (ॐ)

The name designating Him is the sacred syllable **oṁ (ॐ). His name is** praṇavaḥ the verse is discussing the significance of the sacred syllable oṁ (ॐ) as representing the divine or ultimate reality. It may delve into its spiritual, philosophical, or metaphysical implications within the context of the text it belongs to.

Īśvaraḥ is expressed (vācya) by the praṇava, oṁkāra. The relationship between the vācaka (expressive) and vācya (expressed) is fixed and already exists like the relationship between a lamp and its light. The relationship between a word and its meaning is not determined by convention.

Lot can be told about this praṇava mantra. Meaning of praṇava is-always -ever new. All other śabda change; but praṇavaḥ never changes and it is nitya. The word oṁ (ॐ) means Īśvaraḥ only, that is the padam, artham (meaning) etc., question is, whether this connection is a state of constant awareness like dīpa, prakāśa or alignment with profound meaning? this connection is a state of constant awareness like dīpa, prakāśa and is always there by svabhāva. During sṛṣṭi itself, Īśvaraḥ took a saṅkalpa that all each word will have this meaning only.

तज्जपस्तदर्थभावनम्।1.28

तज्-जपस्-तद्-अर्थ-भावनम्।

तज् -(taj)-its, of the syllable oṁ (ॐ)

जपः–(japaḥ)-repetition or recitation of that oṁ (ॐ), the sacred syllable

अर्थ-(artha)- significance

भावनम्-(bhāvanam)- contemplation or meditation, dwelling upon

the repetition or recitation of that praṇava mantra, the sacred syllable with contemplation or meditation on its meaning should be performed.

This sūtrā suggests that the practice of mantra (any mantra- here praṇava) (repetition) should be accompanied by contemplation on its meaning or significance, rather than being merely mechanical repetition.

This adds depth and understanding to the practice, enhancing its spiritual and transformative effects. One must do japa and dhyāna of praṇava and its meaning, namely Īśvaraḥ.

By doing like this āvaraṇa vikṣepa Śakti decreases,

(आवरण (āvaraṇa): Covering or concealing.

विक्षेप(vikṣepa): Distraction or dispersion.

शक्ति (śakti): Power or ability)

(the power or ability to deflect or disperse distractions or disturbances)

(this must be understood like this- distractions will decrease) and yōgis manas attains aikākgriyam (the capability to remain focused or undisturbed despite external influences or distractions) and because of attaining aikākgriyam, a yōgi gets samādhi, and due to this Īśvara prakāśam

ततः प्रत्यक्चेतनाधिगमोऽप्यन्तरायाभावाश्च।1.29

tataḥ pratyak cētanādhigamō' api antarāyābhāvāś ca

ततः-(tataḥ)- thereafter

प्रत्यक्- (pratyak)-inner

चेतना-(cetanā)- consciousness-

अधिगमः-adhigamaḥ-(pratyakchetanādhigamaḥ): direct perception

अपि-(api)-also

अन्तराय-(antarāyā)-interruptions

अभाव- (abhāvāḥ)-absence of obstacles

च-(ca)-also, as well

From this comes the realisation of the inner consciousness and freedom from all disturbances

ब्रह्मनारदीय पुराण- brahmanāradīya purāṇa quotes:

One who wants liberation, the path is only devotion to viṣṇu. Meditate constantly on Him (with His

guṇa and rūpa as in His divya maṅgala vigraha, with manas. He is also the protector. **(रक्षकन्)-for those who have staunch faith in Him, Vishnu reveals Himself in some form, which is different from** prakṛti

Overall, sūtrā emphasizes that through the practice of yōgaḥ, one can attain direct perception (pratyakchetanādhigamaḥ) and overcome obstacles (antarāyābhāvāḥ), suggesting a state of clarity and freedom from hindrances on the path of spiritual realization.

Due to praṇava dhyāna puruṣa's, removal of vighna happens and real svarūpa jñānam is realised.

Due to īśvara prasāda, diseases will move away from him and will not come to him. He will see his real svarūpa. Since puruṣa (one whose buddhi is made prakāśa) has identical guṇa of īśvara, (unlike two vastus which have different guṇas)- namely not having klēsa, janma end, limited āyuś, bhōga, punya and pāpa, puruṣa when he understands one, he will understand another also. Since puruṣa has guṇa same as that of īśvara (called guṇa sāmyam) when he understands īśvara- svarūpa-it automatically means he understands his own svarūpa. Pratyak- cētana is one who does not know the reality but misunderstands the same (vibharīta-diverse or varied). But due to praṇava dhyāna, manas goes towards inside klēsas are removed, obstacles eliminated and he understands own svarūpa correctly.

व्याधिस्त्यानसंशयप्रमादालस्याविरतिभ्रान्तिदर्शनालब्धभूमिकत्वानवस्थितत्वानि चित्तविक्षेपास्तेऽन्तरायाः।1.30

Vyādhi-styāna-saṁśaya-pramādālasyāvirati-bhrānti-darśanālabdha-bhūmikatvānavasthatatvāni-citta-vikṣēpās tē'ntarāyāḥ

व्याधि-(vyādhi) - illness

स्त्यान-(styāna) - mental laziness

संशय-(saṃśaya) - doubt

प्रमाद-(pramāda) - negligence

आलस्य-(ālasya) - sloth

अविरति-(avirati) - lack of detachment

भ्रान्ति-(bhraṃti) – delusion, confusion, error

दर्शन-(darśana) – perception

आलब्ध-(ālabdha) - non-attainment

भूमिकत्व-(bhūmi-katva) – instability, not attaining a base

अनवस्थितत्व-(anavasthatatvāni) - instability, inability to maintain

चित्त (citta) - mind

विक्षेप-(vikṣepa) - distraction

ते-(te) – these, of them

अन्तराय-(**a**ntarāyāḥ) -obstacles

These disturbances are disease, idleness, doubt, carelessness, sloth, (reluctance-to-work) lack of detachment, misapprehension, failure to attain a base for concentration, and instability, they are distractions for the mind. These, disturbances are impurities of yōga, its enemy and obstacles produced by rajas and tamas guṇā.

śankarā says they are called disturbances because they move and make a gap in one's practice.

Disease comes to one because of vāda pitta ślēṣma dhātu, rasam of intake food (āhāra rasam) and senses such as manas lacks integrity, or without honesty.

दुःखदौर्मनस्याङ्गमेजयत्वश्वासप्रश्वासा विक्षेपसहभुवः।1.31

duḥkhadaurmanasyāṅgamējayatvaśvāsapraśvāsā vikṣēpasahabhuvaḥ

Suffering, dejection, trembling, inhalation, and exhalation accompany distractions

दुःख-(duḥkha): suffering

दौर्मनस्य-(daurmanasya): mental distress, dejection

अङ्गमेजयत्व-(aṅgam-ejayatva): restlessness in the limbs

श्वासप्रश्वासा-(śvāsapraśvāsā): irregular breathing

विक्षेप-(vikṣepa): distractions

सहभुवः-(sahabhuva): accompanying

Suffering, mental distress (dejection), restlessness in the limbs, irregular breathing, all accompany distractions. But these distractions do not affect a yōgi, whose mind is fixed. A yōgi has control over mind and so these distractions do not affect them, or cause pain or dejection to them. Ultimately, they all disappear due to devotion to Īśvarā

duḥkha- is a pratikūla-anubhava and due to ādyātmika- (relating to self) ādhibhautika- (related to primary elements or created beings) ādhidaivika- (caused by divine or supernatural agencies)

daurmanasya- is due to efforts going waste and causing mental distress (mana sañcalam)

aṅgamējayatva- Movements of bodily parts. This is an enemy for yōgābhyāsa

śvāsapraśvāsā- breath going in and out freely without one's own power or control. recaka, pūraka etc are allowing śvāsa to take place within certain mātrā. (a mātrā corresponds to a single clap of hands or opening and closing of eyes once. Twelve mātrā are the units used for one cycle of prāṇāyāmaḥ)

तत्प्रतिषेधार्थम् एकतत्त्वाभ्यासः ।1.32

tat-pratiṣēdhārtham ēkatattvābhyāsaḥ

तत्-(tat) -these distractions and their associated accompaniments

प्रतिषेध-(pratiṣedha) -rejection, repel

अर्थम्-(artham) -for the sake of

एक-(eka) -one

तत्त्व-(tattva) -object, principle

अभ्यासः-(abhyāsaḥ)-practice

Practice of fixing the mind on one object performed to eliminate these disturbances- suffering, mental distress, restlessness in the limbs, irregular breathing, tendency to wander towards external objects and to focus it on a single object.

To concentrate on one tattva is to concentrate on īśvara. Any object is also an opinion. But looking at previous sutras, it is best to concentrate on īśvara since we want manas to not oscillate and stay focussed.

मैत्रीकरुणामुदितोपेक्षणांसुखदुःखपुण्यापुण्यविषयाणां भावनातश्चित्तप्रसादनम्।

1.33

Maitri-karuṇā-muditō-pēkṣaṇāṁ-sukha-duḥkha-puṇyā-puṇya-viṣayāṇāṁ-bhāvanātaś-citta-prasādanam

मैत्री-(maitri): Friendship, friendliness

करुणा-(karuna): Compassion

मुदिता-(muditā): Gladness, joy

उपेक्षाणं-(upēkṣaṇāṁ): Equanimity, indifference

सुख-(sukha): Happiness, pleasure

दुःख-(duhkha): Suffering, pain

पुण्य-(punya): Virtue, merit

अपुण्य-(apunya): Vice, demerit

विषयाणां-(vishayanam): Objects, subjects

भावनातूः(bhāvanātaḥ)-attitude

चित्त-(citta): manas, by contemplating upon

प्रसादनम् (prasadanam): Bringing serenity, purification, clarification

This sūtrā, highlights the importance of cultivating positive mental attitudes and equanimity to achieve mental clarity and peace.

This sūtrā, emphasises:

By cultivating an attitude of, friendship towards those who are happy, compassion to those in distress, joy to those virtuous, and equanimity to those non-virtuous, lucidity (intelligibility) arises in mind.

It also prescribes, a mental cultivation, for day-to-day affairs, outside (योगश्चित्तवृत्तिनिरोधः।)

yōgaścittavṛttinirōdhaḥ type meditation. yogic path requires cultivating higher qualities of sattva continuously and constantly because one must face all aspects of life affairs and social interactions. Therefore, this sūtrā, brings out a fact that yōga is to be considered as perfectly in synchronisation with and benevolent to social actions of the normal life.

By doing this (by cultivating an attitude of, friendship towards those who are happy, compassion to those in distress, joy to those virtuous, and equanimity to those non-virtuous,) manas gets steady, becomes pure and rajas, tamas guṇa are eliminated, attains sattva guṇa. citta attains aikākgriyam and mind stops oscillation and remains focussed on īśvara

प्रच्छर्दन-विधारणाभ्यां वा प्राणस्य।1.34

pracchardana-vidhāraṇābhyāṁ- vā- praṇasya.

प्रच्छर्दन-by exhaling

विधारणाभ्यां-by retention

वा or

प्राणस्य--of the breath

Stability of mind is gained by exhaling and retaining the breath. By breathing techniques, body becomes light, and mind turns steady. Since mind is connected to breath directly, by subduing breath, mind is subdued. That is how one attains steadiness of mind and focus on one point(concentration). Therefore, practice meditation with breath control and then only mind becomes free from vrittis and approach SamAdhi state, otherwise mind is disturbed

This sūtrā gives many revelations.

1. patañjali muni has already presented īśvarā as the object of concentration by recitation of praṇavamantrā oṁ (ॐ). Many sūtrā, dedicate īśvarā first in the list (prioritised No 1)
2. vā in this sūtrā and following sūtrā are all alternate techniques for fixing the mind.
3. śankarā says in his bāṣya, one or more techniques(options) might be more suitable to a particular person, time, and place
4. In this sūtrā patañjali muni gives another option CONTROL of breath, for fixing the mind through control of prāṇa
5. However friendliness, compassion etc stated in 1.33 must be cultivated for all instances.

   exhalation, (pracardana) says vyāsa bhāṣya, is expulsion of stomach air through nostrils by special techniques and retention is restraint of breath.
6. Slowing the exhalation and lengthening the retention of the prāṇa within the body is the key
7. Inhalation is a natural process and hence not mentioned in this sūtrā. breath control prāṇāyāma, is specifically brought out in this sūtrā, for gaining control of mind. This is for advanced practitioner of yoga
8. During exhalation and retention of breath, nerves of the body relax. If chest and body are kept still, then only abdominal muscles take control of breath control. Then after abhyāsa retention and exhalation takes place effortlessly requiring no separate effort for kumbakā, and recakā. This leads to, (after prolonged practice) lightness of the body, a happy feeling.

மன்மனமேங்குண்டுவாயுவு மங்குண்டு

மன்மனமெங்கில்லை வாயுவு மங்கில்லை

மன்மனத்துள்ளே மகிழ்திருப் பார்க்கு

மன்மனத்துள்ளே மனோலய மாமே (திரு மந்திரம்)

Exhalation and restraining (holding breath inside) are stated in this sutra. That is without doing pūraka, carrying out kumbhaka. That is allowing the breath which went out to stay outside only. By doing like this body becomes light(laghutva). After this manas becomes steady (stira). Pūraka, kumbhaka, and rēcaka is different method which is not stated in this sūtra.

विषयवती वा प्रवृत्तिरुत्पन्ना मनसः स्थितिनिबन्धनी।1.35

viṣayavatī vā pravr̥ttir utpannā manasaḥ sthiti nibandhanī

विषयवती (viṣayavatī) – containing a sense object

वा (vā) - or

प्रवृत्तिः(pravṛttiḥ) - activity

उत्पन्ना (utpannā) - arises

मनसः(manasaḥ) - of the mind

स्थिति (sthiti) – state

निबन्धनि (nibandhanī)

in bondage, causing steadiness

or else focus on the sense object arises and this causes steadiness of the mind on viṣaya

This sūtrā suggests that when the mind is caught up in external objects (or when there is activity arising), it indicates bondage of the mind.

This is a tricky sūtrā needs a bit of explanation. Let us see the explain.

While viṣaya could refer to any sense object, vyāsā comments in this sūtra that viṣaya could be connected to supersensuous experiences. It is stated by him **that if one concentrate, on the tip of the nose, one could experience a divine or a supernormal sense of smell. On the tip of the tongue a super normal taste, and on the root of the tongue**

a super normal sound etc. These experiences fix the mind, eliminate doubt, and leads one to samādhi state. Note that patañjali muni has used "manas" here instead of **citta**, because traditionally **"citta"** interacts with senses directly and here we talk of supersensuous experiences.

It is to be noted that sense object can be used as a support for the manas. It is also to be noted here that oṁ (ॐ) meditation can be audible and it would act as a help, and since as long as manas is fixed on it, it does not matter. This is contradictory to conventional or traditional teachings.

vyāsā says, even though, true nature of reality is known through scriptures, inferences (pratyakṣa anumāna and śabda) or through a guru, if one does not experience these higher realities, personally through one's own senses, it (that knowledge) remains second hand only. This is fundamental for believing Liberation per-se. Therefore, if a sādhaka, can experience one of the above stated, supernormal feelings through senses, then faith in scriptures would improve, and increase and therefore, strengthened. One's manas believes that sūkṣmaviśaya are indeed true. This is why manas is given samskāra abhyāsa practice. Since vr̥tti keep changing very fast, in order to restrain those vr̥ttis, lot of abhyāsa are taught (given to manas). If those abhyāsa must be useful i.e. manas must become steady and stable, one must develop vairāgya in other viṣaya and that is called vaśīkāra

More specifically faith in **īśvarā** is strengthened and so, the faith in ability to concentrate on **īśvarā**. These type of concentration needs to be practiced continuously for a longer period, while fasting or minimal diet and in a quiet place where no disturbances occur.

विशोका वा ज्योतिष्मती।1.36

viśōkā vā jyōtiṣmatī

विशोका-(Viśokā): Without grief, painless

वा-(vā) or

ज्योतिष्-(jyotiṣ): luminous, effulgent

मति-(matī): possessing

Or steadiness of manas is attained when manas is pain free and luminous ((luminous-full knowledge)

This sūtrā highlights the potential experiences and states of being that can be attained through yōgic practices. One is a state free from sorrow or grief, indicating a state of inner peace and tranquillity, and the other is a state illuminated by inner light, symbolizing a higher state of consciousness or enlightenment.

patañjali muni in this sūtrā states, one must free himself from rajas and tamas, which are sources of pain and ignorance. sattva is luminous (illumination of knowledge) and blissful (ānanda-mayā) by svabhāva (nature).

Contemplating on ātmā in this state, ego loses awareness of any other object and is aware only of ātmā without attributing importance to " ātmā ".

This course is not the ultimate goal of yōga. This is the base for perceiving **īśvarā**

Let us see how gītācārya (Lord kṛṣṇā says in bhagavadgītā) gives lakṣaṇa for ātmasātkṣātkāra

यत् ज्ञात्वा न पुनर्मोहमेवं यास्यसि पाण्डव।

येन भूतान्यशेषेण द्रक्ष्यस्यात्मन्यथो मयि।।(BG 4.35)

The way you will not attain moha (desire) by attaining such ज्ञानम्- knowledge and with same ज्ञानम् see all ātmā including tiryak (animals etc) in you and then see them all in me that is ātmasātkṣātkāra

Here you (any ātmā) will see me (īśvarā) in you, is the right interpretation. This ज्ञानम् is earned through śikṣā, through a guru who has done ātmasātkṣātkāra, and carrying out karma- yōga as bhagavadārādhanam and with three tyāga. (kartr̥tva, mamatā, and phala)

If one, stabilises his manas in heart (hradaya) and carry out dhāraṇa, dhyāna, and samādhi buddhi becomes nirmala and spreads everywhere like ākāśam. heart (hradaya) has a cakra. That is in the adhōmukha state. By parāṇāyāma, one must turn it ūrdhvamukha state and focus manas there. That is the right place for manas. When manas is focussed here all planets, sun, moon, and (gems) ratna are visible as light. This state is spoken in this sūtrā as jyotiṣmatī. Here a yōgi's manas become stable and steady.

वीतरागविषयं वा चित्तम्।1.37

vītarāgaviṣayaṁ vā cittam

वीत-(vīta)-without

राग-(rāga): attachment, desire

विषयं-(viṣayaṁ): towards objects

वा-(vā): or

चित्तम्-(cittam): the mind

When the mind is free from desire(attachment) to objects it becomes steady (निश्चलम्)

However, vyāsā who wrote commentary has different view on this sūtrā. He says the goal of yōga can be attained by meditation by a pure minded yōgi. When contemplating the mind on those pure minded yōgis, (one who is free from desire), one's own mind becomes pure by their association

(Here, bhajagovindam by ādi śankara could be quoted)

सत्सङ्गत्वे निस्सङ्गत्वं.....bhajagovindam

satsaṅgatve nissaṅgatvam

सत्सङ्गत्वे-(satsaṅgatve)-in the company of the virtuous or in the association of good people. निस्सङ्गत्वम्-(nissaṅgatvam)-absence of association or disassociation

So, the phrase "सत्सङ्गत्वे निस्सङ्गत्वम्" can be translated to "In the company of the virtuous, there is disassociation," or more generally, "association with good company leads to detachment."

This phrase emphasizes the influence of one's surroundings and the importance of surrounding oneself with virtuous or good people to cultivate detachment from worldly distractions and attachments Through association with the wise, there arises non-attachment.

By association with such persons, we have also raised in our level of selflessness and compassion, if not got rid of desire. One gets affected by the company one keeps. This sūtrā points out the guru-śiṣya(relationships) or lineage recommended by our scriptures. bhagavadgītā also quotes in 4.34,

तत् विद्धि प्रणिपातेन परिप्रश्नेन सेवया।

उपदेक्ष्यन्ति ते ज्ञानम् ज्ञानिनस्तत्वदर्शिनः।।(BG 4.34)

by intense dedication and service to a yōgi with pure sattvic mind and learning from him, one's own mind can become steady (niścalam) and free from personal desires (detachment to worldly pleasures).

Many of our scriptures recommend, total surrender and service to the guru as the highest form of meditation (dhyāna)

In summary, freedom from desire and tranquillity are minimum qualities one must have who says "I have realised self and Īśvarā within.bhagavadgītāstressesthepointthatanger,detachment(freeof desire)arenon-negotiableforayōgi.Sameistaughtbypatañjalimuni in many sūtrā where yama and niyama are spoken by him.

स्वप्निनिद्राज्ञानालंबनं वा।1.38

svapninidrājñānālaṁbanaṁ vā

or mind can become steady when knowledge attained from sleep and dream as its support. Another meaning is that in dream and sleep do not let jñāna "I" slip away from you.

When one goes from waking to sleep state or sleep to deep sleep (suṣupti) the connection to prajñā "I" is cut. That connection should not get cut and prajñā "I" must continue. One should strive to move away from this loss. That is the aim of this sūtrā.

swapna -When senses do not have any viṣaya, and manas is having vāsanā rūpa anubhava, that is the state of swapna. In swapna if a mahān, or dēvatā appears and if one focusses the manas on them, **yōgi's** manas becomes steady or focussed, and perseverance.

suṣupti- I slept well is the only jñānam of sattvika suṣupti which will be come in memory(smr̥ti). In that state, (nidrā state in which sukha anubhava was experienced,) manas will be in its own state. That is ēkāgram (concentration, undisturbed stage) state. Those who are brahmavids, say that this sukha itself is brahma svarūpa. One must note the discussion about suṣupti in chāndōgya upaniṣad

स्वप्न-(swapna)-dream

निद्रा-(nidrā) -sleep

ज्ञान-(jñāna) -knowledge

आलंबनं-(ālambanaṁ) -support, dependent on

वा (vā) -or

This sūtrā suggests that certain types of knowledge or experiences may arise from dreams or deep sleep states. It implies that understanding can come from sources beyond waking consciousness, highlighting the potential for insights gained during dream or deep meditation states.

यथाभिमतद्यानाद् वा।1.39

yatābhimatadyānād vā

यत-(yata) – according to, which, whatever

अभिमत-(abhimata) – that which is agreeable, desired, pleasing

ध्यानात्-(dhyānāt) – for meditation

वा-(vā) - or

Or steadiness of mind can be attained from meditation upon whatever object (of anything) of one's inclination (or principle one finds uplifting or pleasing)

This sūtrā suggests that a person can achieve a state of inner peace or concentration (which is essential for progressing in yōga) by meditating on whatever object or principle they find inspiring or enjoyable. It emphasizes the flexibility and personalization of meditation practices. This **sūtrā** is part of the section that describes various methods for achieving the concentration of the mind, highlighting that the path to inner tranquillity and the focused state of yōga can be individualized based on what best resonates with the practitioner.

If one concentrates on anything which he likes, (dharmic things only) manas will stay on that. i.e. (focus on that) and because of this one will attain ēkāgram. If a dēvatā is focussed on dhyana in the most liked roopa, a **yōgi will attain sthairyam (steadfastness or stability, perseverance)**

परमाणुपरममहत्त्वान्तोऽस्य वशीकारः।1.40;

paramāṇuparamamahatvānto'sya vaśīkāraḥ

The yōgi's mastery extends from the smallest particle of matter, to the ultimate totality of matter

परम-(parama)-greatest, finest, most distinguished

अणु-(aṇu)-atom

परम-(parama)-ultimate

महत्व-(mahatva)-totality of matter,प्रकृति-prakṛti)

अन्तः-(antaḥ)-up to

अस्य-(asya)-the yogi's

वशीकारः-(vaśīkāraḥ)-mastery

This sūtrā suggests, that the mind of a yōgi becomes so refined and concentrated that he can gain mastery or control from the smallest entity (atom) to the largest or the ultimate in magnitude प्रकृति-prakṛti)). It highlights the depth and the expansive capacity of the mind through the practice of yōga. It indicates that through practice and discipline, a person can control their mind to such an extent that it can understand

and connect with entities ranging from the most minute to the largest. mind is all pervading and underpins all physical forms. It can pervade any form or dimension and assumes that form's shape and quality. By such mastery, a yōgi bypasses the need for everything since nothing can obstruct a yōgi who has mastery over his mind. śankarā says "after obtaining this" a yōgi travels to samādhi state. A yōgi who has attained this state gets ēkāgram need not practice further to attain this state.

क्षीणवृत्तेरभिजातस्येव मणेर्ग्रहीतृग्रहणग्राह्येषु

तत्स्थ तदञ्जनतासमापत्ति।।1.41

kṣīṇavṛtterabhijātasyeva maṇergrahītṛgrahaṇagrāhyeṣu

tatstha tadañjanatāsamāpatti

क्षीण-(kṣīṇa)-weekened

वृत्तेः-(vṛtteḥ)-fluctuating states of mind

अभिजातस्य-(abhijātasya)- transparent

इव-(iva)-like

मणेः(maṇeḥ)- of a jewel

ग्रहीतृ-(grahītṛ)-the knower

ग्रहण-(grahaṇa)-the instrument of knowledge

ग्राह्येषु-(grāhyeṣu)-in the object of knowledge

तत्-(tat)-that

स्थ-(stha)- situated

तत्-(tat)-that

अञ्जनता-(añjanatā)-influenced- taking the form of

समापत्तिः-(samāpattiḥ)- complete absorption of an object

samāpattiḥ, complete absorption of mind when it is free from its vṛttis occurs when the mind becomes like a transparent jewel(crystal) taking the form of whatever object is placed before it, whether the object is the knower, the instrument of knowledge, or the object of knowledge.

When the fluctuations of the mind are calmed down and the mind becomes clear like a crystal, the yōgi achieves a state of complete absorption (samādhi), wherein the knower (the seer), the act of knowing (perception), and the known (the perceivable) become like one. In this state, the mind becomes as transparent as a gem and assumes the colour or the form of whatever it focuses on, whether it is the object of concentration or the self, indicating a seamless unity between the subject, the process of perception, and the object.

This sūtrā describes a high level of mental clarity and concentration where the mind is so pure and undisturbed that it reflects whatever it perceives without distortion, just as a perfectly clear crystal reflects the colour of whatever object is placed near it.

vṛttis are three types-sattva, rajas and tamas. rajas and tamas decay where as sattva remains when manas is placed near a sphaṭika (crystal) as seen earlier. Manas takes sattva vṛttis inside and the other two goes out of manas. To start with these two rajas and tamas decay and manas starts to see inside and only sattva vṛttis exist. Later this also will decay. When in manas rajas, tamas vṛttis are there manas would be weak and impure. When these decay and sattva vṛttis increase manas would become like a sphaṭika (crystal) and attain nirmala state. That time whichever vastu to which manas is associated, it becomes the same vastu. This is called grāhyasamāpatti. (yield to-coming together) this is one state. Second is when manas does not associate with viṣaya, but only associate with senses and take them as viṣaya. Third is when manas is associated only with ātmā. This is called grahaṇasamāpatti (grahaṇa means senses) or grahītirusamāpatti. (meaning for this word grahītiru is one who is seizing- ātmā). In addition to ātmā, making manas depended on self, concentrating with manas on prahlada, sukhar etc also., samāpatti

तत्र शब्दार्थज्ञानविकल्पैःसंकीर्णा सवितर्का समापत्तिः ।1.42

tatra śabdārthajñānavikalpaiḥsaṁkīrṇā savitarkā samāpattiḥ

in this stage, savitarkāsamāpattiḥ samādhi absorption with physical awareness inter-mixed with notions of word, meaning and idea.

तत्र-(tatra) = there, in that

शब्द-(śabda) = word, sound

अर्थ-(artha) = meaning

ज्ञान-(jñāna) = knowledge

विकल्पैः-(vikalpaiḥ) = with conceptualisation, with alternatives, with options,

संकीर्णा-(saṁkīrṇā) = mixed with

सवितर्का-(savitarkā) = with physical awareness, with deliberation, with argumentation

समापत्तिः-(samāpattiḥ) = absorption, engrossment, deep understanding

The state of savitarkā samāpattiḥ (absorption with deliberation) is that in which, knowledge of the object is mixed with word, and its meaning, and is accompanied by conceptualization. In yōga direct perception is the highest means of gaining knowledge, and so, one must practice and experience the truths of yōga, not merely theoretically, but must try and understand the meaning also.

This refers to a state of consciousness where the yōgi's mind is absorbed in an object of meditation, but this absorption still involves some level of conceptual thinking or analysis. The yōgi is aware of the object through its name, meaning, and the knowledge that arises from it, but there is still a distinction between the object, its name, and the associated knowledge. This is considered an initial or preliminary stage of deeper meditative absorption, leading towards more profound states of samādhi where such distinctions eventually dissolve.

vyāsā explains this as follows:

A yōgi's understanding of an object is mixed with awareness of what the object is called and the memory or idea corresponding to that object. According to this sūtrā, the experience of the object is mixed up (saṁkīrṇā) with vikalpa i.e. mental images with alternatives in the form of words and ideas. Therefore, direct experience of the object is tainted by the imposition of conceptual thought on it. The yōgi should not deliberate or reason out about the object in any kind of analysis, and use intellect for the thought of understanding. Nor a yōgi should consciously activate a saṁskāra to recognise the object since that would mean mental vr̥ttis. But a yōgi at samādhi stage is one whose vr̥ttis are stilled. He further states that "the perception of the true nature of the object gained through samāpattiḥ is the best. Here the comparison to a yōgi is like this: nirvitarkā samāpattiḥ is direct perception that transcends words, and ideas and gives the essential nature of an object, at a more profound level of word, meaning and idea. This is called as para pratyakṣā (super-perception) than loka-pratyakṣā (mundane perception) by him. In other words, yōgi who has attained this stage of samādhi, use word and logic which become the base for scriptures., nirvitarkā awareness of reality is expressed by īśvarā or yōgis who have attained this type of samādhi, through words and concepts.

स्मृतिपरिशुद्धौ स्वरूपशून्येवार्थ मात्रनिर्भासा निर्वितर्का।1.43

smṛtipariśuddhausvarūpaśūnyevārthamātranirbhāsā nirvartakā.

स्मृति-(smṛti)-memory

परिशुद्धौ-(pariśuddhau)-Upon purification of memory, termination of memory

स्वरूप-(svarūpa)-own nature/form

शून्य-(śūnya)-devoid of its

इव-(iva)-as if

अर्थ-(artha)-object, meaning

मात्र-(mātra)-only

निर्भासा-(nirbhāsā)-shines forth, appears

निर्वितर्का- (nirvitarkāḥ)-without physical awareness, without deliberation/thought

Patanjali Muni discusses in this Sūtrā, a state of consciousness where, upon the purification of memory (freeing the mind from past impressions), the object of focus appears devoid of its own nature and shines forth in its purest form, unmingled with the mind's own projections or deliberations. This state is referred to as "nirvitarka samapatti," a type of samadhi (deep absorption) where the mind is completely absorbed in the essence of the object of meditation without the interference of subjective perception or thought. This level of clarity and purity in perception occurs when the mind is free from the distortions of personal memory and bias, allowing the object to be perceived in its true essence.

Nirvitarka-samāpatti- "absorption without conceptualisation" occurs when memory is completely purged and the mind is

empty, as it were, of its own nature. In this state only the object of meditation shines forth. When one has attained this stage, (individual has purged all samaṁsārik memories to understand the object of meditation). one loses an attachment to family, wealth etc and could focus on the object.

nirvitarka samāpatti- After one loses smṛti, and stays as if "I" prajñā is not there, and remains like a vastu under dhyāna. In this **samāpatti-** thought of experience undergone through, smṛti, pratayakṣam, śabdam, and anumāna pramāṇam is not there, and manas becomes vastu rūpa itself. This samāpatti is to do dhyāna on stūla vastu

एतयैव सविचारा निर्विचरा च सूक्ष्मविषया व्याख्याता।1.44

Etayaiva savicārā nirvicarā ca sūkṣma-viṣayā vyākhyātā

एतय-(etaya)-by this very (method); implying the same method as previously discussed

सविचारा-(savicārā)-with subtle thought; reflective, deliberative

निर्विचरा-(nirvicārā)-without subtle thought; super reflective, non-deliberative

च (ca)-and

सूक्ष्म-(sūkṣma)-subtle

विषया-(viṣayā)-objects

व्याख्याता-(vyākhyātā)- are explained; are described

The states of samādhi with/without subtle awareness, and whose objects of focus are subtle in nature are explained in the same manner

This sūtrā continues the discussion on the types of (samādhi, meditative absorption) and explains that by the same method (as discussed in the previous sūtrā related to saṁprajñāta-samādhi and the objects of meditation, the states of meditation with subtle thought (savicāra) and without subtle thought (nirvicāra), both concerning subtle objects, are explained, or described.

Essentially, patañjali muni is elaborating on the stages of concentration that lead one towards deeper meditative states, focusing on more subtle objects of meditation, moving from a state where there is still some form of contemplation or thought (savicāra) to a state where even those subtle thoughts cease (nirvicāra), aiming towards pure awareness or consciousness without an object of focus.

patañjali muni says सविचार (savicāra), निर्विचार (nirvicāra) as it is in Sanskrit, since English translations of the same is incomprehensible. satvitarka-samāpatti and nirvitarka-samāpatti represent stoola objects and concentrate on gross physical objects, whereas savicāra and nir-nirvicāra concentrate on sūkṣma objects (subtle objects). It is also defined that gross elements are evolved from subtle elements and so, subtle aspects cannot be perceived by the gross senses. Subtler things can only be perceived by things even subtler than themselves. Here the concept of tanmātrā is introduced. It is to be noted that subtle elements (sound, touch, taste, sight, smell-panca tanmātrā are the sources from which gross elements evolve. This is what is perceived in savicāra samādhi. vicāra then is meditative focus, becomes absorbed in tanmātrā, the subtle elements underpinning any object of meditation. Then a **yōgi** goes to a nirvicāra state where he transcends time and space, and perceive these subtle essences, pervade, and always underpin all things.

In the higher states of samādhi, tanmātrā are not only subtle elements, but they themselves are evolutes still subtler entities such as ahaṁkāra and buddhi. These subtler elements can also be object of samādhi

Vicāra is one stage of dhyāna and not tarka vicāra (reasoning). sūkṣma vastu means parama aṇu. These are methods to stop oscillations of manas

सूक्ष्मविषयत्वं चालिङगपर्यवसानम्।1.45

sūkṣma viṣayatvaṁ cāliṅga-paryavasānam

सूक्ष्म-(sūkṣma)-subtle

विषयत्वं-(viṣayatvaṃ)-subtleness of the object, things having the nature of

च (ca)-and

आलिङ्ग-(āliṅga)- prakr̥ti that which has no sign

पर्यवसानम्-(paryavasānam)-terminate, this gives the extent to which the understanding can go.

prakr̥ti is the ultimate subtler cause of everything because nothing is subtler than this.

The subtleness of the object indicates the end. This verse, from patañjali muni, suggests that when one's attention becomes extremely refined and focused on an object during meditation (subtleness of the object), it signifies the culmination or the nearing of the end of that meditative state or process.

As one approach more subtler levels of prakr̥ti, sattva element becomes dominant. One of the inherent qualities of sattva is ānanda. A yōgi first reaches this ānanda state (sattvic aspect of prakr̥ti) which is different from ānanda of brahmam stated in upaniṣad. Finally, a yōgi reaches a state of reality the subtlest nature "buddhi"

puruṣa the jīvā is changeless according to yōga school and does not produce anything grosser than itself. patañjali muni does not connect īśvarā as the material cause of the universe

ता एव सबीजःसमाधिः।1.46

tā ēva sa-bījaḥ samādhiḥ

ता-(tā)- those (referring back to the types of samadhi mentioned in previous sūtrās)

एव-(eva) = only, just, indeed

सबीज-(sabījaḥ)- with seed; sabījaḥ, here refers to samadhi that still **has an object of focus**, which acts as the **'seed'** for concentration.

समाधिः(samādhi)-a state of intense concentration or meditative absorption.

The above-mentioned samāpatti states are known as samādhiḥ (meditative absorption) with seed" "sabījaḥ samādhiḥ". This implies that in these states of samādhiḥ, there is still an object of meditation or focus that the mind holds onto, which acts as the 'seed' for concentration

This sūtrā is part of patañjali muni's explanation of the different levels of samādhi (meditative absorption) and can be translated to mean "those only are samādhi with seed." In other words, the types of samādhi mentioned up to this point in the yōg-sūtrā are considered " sa-bīja samadhi", or samādhi with seed. This implies that in these states of samādhi, there is still an object of meditation or focus that the mind holds onto, which acts as the 'seed' for concentration. This contrasts with nir-bīja samādhi, which is a state of samādhi without an object of focus, where the mind is completely absorbed, free from the duality of subject and object.

All four samādhi explained above are with bīja which means there is still an object of meditation or focus that the mind holds onto, and that acts as the 'seed' for concentration.

निर्विचारवैशारद्येऽध्यात्मप्रसादः ।।1.47

nirvicāravaiśāradyē'dhyātmaprasādaḥ

निर्विचार-(nirvicāra)- reflection or discrimination;

वैशारद्ये-(vaiśāradye)- clarity

अध्यात्म-(adhyātma)-of inner self

प्रसादः-(prasādaḥ): lucidity of the Self

Upon attaining the clarity of nirvicāra-samādhi there is lucidity of the inner self.

This phrase indicates that spiritual realization comes not through intellectual analysis but through the grace of the self.

rajas and tamas create a situation of hiding viṣaya. Because these are removed by yogābhyāsa, manas brightens as sattva. Normally, for other people jñānam comes one by one in order. But for those who reach this state all viṣaya jñānam is reached at once, at one time (for a yōgi). This person sees all other with extreme compassion(empathy).

ऋतंभरा तत्र प्रज्ञा ।1.48

r̥taṁ bharā tatra prajñā

ऋतं-(ṛtaṁ) Filled with truth or reality, cosmic order

भरा-(bharā)-bearing or filled with

तत्र-(tatra)-there, in that place or state.

प्रज्ञा-(prajñā)-wisdom or higher knowledge.

In that state, there is truth-bearing wisdom.

There, in that state, wisdom is filled with truth (or reality, cosmic order).

This sūtrā refers to a state of deep, meditative absorption (samādhi) where the wisdom or knowledge that arises is no longer based on empirical evidence or logical inference, but is direct, intuitive, and filled with the ultimate truth of reality. This wisdom transcends the limitations of ordinary perception and intellectual understanding, being rooted in direct, experiential knowledge of the true nature of existence.

It is difficult to comprehend. A subtle thing can be understood only by another subtler thing. No doubt ātma is subtle; but since Īśvara is subtler and pervades every ātma how can one realise the same in būloka? will see any explanations in the coming sūtrās.

श्रुतानुमानप्रज्ञाभ्याम् अन्यविषया विशेषार्थत्वात्।1.49

Śrutānumāna-prajñābhyām anya-viṣayā viśēṣā arthatvāt

1. श्रुत-(Śruta) -Heard or scriptural knowledge, refers to knowledge acquired through listening or studying texts.
2. अनुमान-(Anumāna) -Inference, knowledge gained through logical reasoning or deduction.
3. प्रज्ञाभ्याम्-(Prajñābhyām)- From/with wisdom, referring to knowledge obtained through profound insight or enlightenment. distinct from, but considered in conjunction with, śruta (scriptural knowledge) and anumāna (inference).

अन्य-(Anya) another, different

विषया-(viṣayā) - object implying that the knowledge in question pertains to a different or special object of understanding, not covered by the earlier mentioned types of knowledge

विशेष-(viśeṣa)-special, particular, specific

अर्थत्वात्-(arthatvāt) - as its object

It (seedless samādhi) has a different focus from that of inference and sacred scripture, because it has particualirity of things as its object

This sūtrā conveys that the knowledge gained through direct spiritual experience (prajñā) is of a different category and pertains to a special subject matter that cannot be accessed through the conventional means of scriptural study (śruta) or inference (anumāna). This type of knowledge is direct, experiential insight into the true nature of reality, which transcends and is more profound than the knowledge gained through external sources or logical deduction. It highlights the uniqueness and superiority of spiritual insight gained through yogic practice, emphasizing that such insight provides a direct, intuitive understanding of the ultimate reality, distinct from the intellectual understanding derived from scriptures or reasoning.

Knowledge gained by śruti and anumāna is of ordinary type. It does not show special qualities of vastus. ṛtaṁ bharā is different. It can enter where śruti and anumāna cannot. By this reality is known and one gets a real jñānam. Here one can get jñānam about sūkṣma parama aṇu, hidden and faraway vastus come in front. These are extraneous to laukīka pratyakṣa, anumāna, and śabda pramāṇā

तज्जः संस्कारोऽन्यसंस्कार प्रतिबन्धी।1.50

tajjaḥ saṁskārō'nyasaṁskāra pratibandhī

तत्-(tat)-that, arising from that

जः–(jaḥ)-born

संस्कारः-(saṁskāraḥ) -subconscious impressions

अन्य-(anya) = other

संस्कार-(saṁskāra) = subconscious impressions

प्रतिबन्धी-(pratibandhī) = inhibiting; obstructing; preventing

The saṁskāras (impressions) born from that [truth bearing wisdom-experience of nirbīja samādhi] obstruct or prevent the formation of other saṁskāras impressions.

This sūtrā emphasizes the transformative power of the experience of nirbīja-samādhi, a state of samādhi without an object of focus, which leads to the highest state of consciousness and enlightenment. The saṁskārā or subconscious impressions created from this profound experience are so potent that they can inhibit or prevent the formation of other, lesser saṁskārā that are the result of ordinary experiences. Essentially, the deep, spiritual insights and understandings gained during such states of samādhi have the power to overshadow and nullify the influences of worldly impressions, steering the practitioner towards liberation (mokṣā) and a state of inner peace and enlightenment.

The saṁskārā born out of that wisdom obstruct other saṁskārā from even emerging in thought

This sūtrā brings out a clear fact that already activated karma of yōgi's present life experience, life span, type of body, ongoing experience are terminated:

ONLY UPON THE MANIFESTATION OF nirbīja-samādhi

A yōgi who attained this state, will not permit external viṣayā to stay in his manas. Even if pūrva vāsanā of that type exist, he will not permit them to take control of his manas. Due to samādhi, prajñā gets stable and steady(stira). Because of this action of samādhi, improves further. In ordinary matters mind stays on them, similarly in samādhi state also mind stays in samādhi to strengthen the same. Both are different. aikākgriyam due to samādhi removes mental viṣayā vāsanā and purifies the manas. Also helps in attaining puruṣa sātkṣātkāra.

Because of attaining puruṣa sātkṣātkāra manas calms down without vṛddhi. mano nāsam(perish) happens. But if manas which gets into viṣayā aikākgriyam, it keeps expanding that experience.

तस्यापि विरोधे सर्वनिरोधान् निर्बीजः समाधिः I1.51

tasyapi virōdhē sarvanirōdhān nirbījaḥ samādhiḥ

तस्य-(tasya) - of that

अपि-(api) - also

निरोधे-(virodhe) - in opposition

सर्व-(sarva) – all

निरोधात्-(nirodhāt) - restraints

निर्बीज-(nirbīja) – seedless, समाधिः-(samādhiḥ) - absorption

Upon the cessation of even those truth bearing saṁskārā nirbīja-samādhi, seedless meditative absorption, ensues

Even in the face of opposition, absorption without seeds (**nirbīja samādhi**) is the culmination of all restraints. **nirbīja-samādhi,** afflicts all saṁskāra. Because of these experiences of viṣayā of mind stops. A yōgi attains kaivalya. In that state a puruṣa is pure and in his own svarūpa. In this state he is called a muktha.in the beginning due to many vṛttis his manas was like a wave in an ocean. Then due to yogabhyāsa many vṛttis are avoided and only one vṛtti stayed. In this state "I" prajñā was there. **After some practice this also vanished and a yōgi attains kaivalya. Note the Tiru-Mantiram given below.**

நானென்றுந் தானென்று நாடிநான் சாரவே

தானென்று நானென் றிலாத் தற்பதந்

தானென்று நானென்ற தத்வ நல்கலாற்

றானென்று நானென்றுஞ் சாற்றகி லேனே (திரு மந்திரம்)

इति पतञ्जलिविरचिते योगसूत्रेप्रतमः समाधिपादः।

Thus ends the first chapter on samādhi, in the yōgaḥ sūtrā composed by **patañjali muni.**

BIBLIOGRAPHY

1. Sanskrit for Shastra study-CIF online classes by Dr. Ved Chaitanya
2. The yogaḥ sūtrā of Patañjali- A new edition, Translation, and Commentary (with insights from the Traditional Commentators)- by Edwin F. Bryant
3. Patañjali yogaḥ sūtram by Brahmaśrī Narayana Iyer -அக்கிராசனாதிபதி (akkirācanādhipati) (the head of the institution) of Madurai Brahma Jñāna Sabhā
4. Bhagavatagītā Tamil vyākyāṇam (gītā sāram) with svāmi deśikan's tātparya candrikā by abhinava deśika śrī. Uttamur veerarghavachariar
5. Internet sources

ABOUT THE AUTHOR

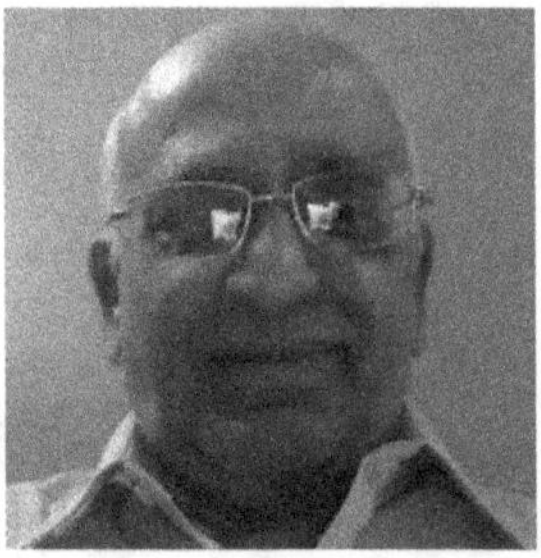

- BE(HONS) ELECTRICAL FROM REC TRICHY YEAR 1971
- M.A. ASTROLOGY (SASTRA UNIVERSITY, TANJORE)- 2019
- PhD (Vedic Astrology) Yoga Samskrutam University (YSAM) Florida, USA-an American Religion University
- Diploma in Sanskrit (Madras Sanskrit college)
- Certificate course in Vedic studies – (Jagat guru Sri Devanath institute of Vedic Science and Research-Nagpur) - Registered center - kavikulaguru Kalidoss Sanskrit University- Nagpur

Various other online course participation and certificates:

- Samvada Suktas online camp - Jan2023- 6 days - Chinmaya International
- Bharatiya Darsana - An Introduction to Indian Philosophical systems-Chinmaya
- Viswavidyapeeth – June&July 2020

- Online Handson Experience on Research Methodology and Biostatistics-Level-2 -Morajidesai National Institute of Yoga, New Delhi July 2020
- How to write a Literature Review Article-Method simplify.com-Sep 2020
- Statistical Analysis using SPSS-Aug 2020-Manonmaniam Sundaranar University, Tirunelveli
- Nyaya, Mimamsa, and Vedanta course conducted by Velukkudi Sri. Ranganathan-2021
- Siksha by Dr. Korada Subrahmanyam Professor of Sanskrit Hyderabad 500 019
- Tantra Yukti -Indica by Dr. Mahadevan

Grantha Catustaya Kalakshepam from Astana Vidwans of Sri Ahibila Mutt:

- Sri.Mannarkudi Rajagopalachariar
- Sri.ThayyarLakshminrasimha charier
- **Samashrayanam done by 44th Azagiya singar and Prapatti done by 45th Azagiya singar**
- **Nrasimha Anushtup Mantropadesam received from 45th Azagiya singar**

Miscellaneous Experiences – Classes, course Guidances on a regular basis

- Taking classes on Bagavat Gita, Vishnu Sahasranamam, SriBhashyam and Rahasya Traya Sara to selected family and friends (Weekly once)
- Taking Astrology classes online to those who need my help
- Guided for Research (PhD) in Marriage breakages - An empirical study by Sri. Ramki Murugan for his ICAS thesis (2023)
- Mr. Gururajan, a colleague of mine in Sastra University who did a PhD in Navamsa at Vel's University Chennai (2023)

- Learning Astrology from different Gurus, Sri. NVRA Raja (Nakshatra Siddhanta)
- Sri. Mantracalam, (Tamil Astrology which he learnt from His Guru-in a Gurukulam for 15 years, Sri. Gayatri Sankar, - Navamsa prediction techniques, ICAS-Chennai Chapter.

Author of three books (published):

- Bramha vidya -Vol-1,
- Bramha vidya -Vol-2
- Yogic Life style for Modern women- On March 8th 2023
  co-Authored for Dr. T Gargi Urmila

www.ingramcontent.com/pod-product-compliance
Lightning Source LLC
LaVergne TN
LVHW010604070526
838199LV00063BA/5068
* 9 7 8 9 3 5 6 4 8 6 4 8 5 *